# LEARNING MEDICINE

## An Evidence-Based Guide

Peter Wei | Alexander Chamessian

Learning Medicine – An Evidence-Based Guide

Cover Design by ShanYi Zhao
Interior Layout by Steven W. Booth, www.GeniusBookServices.com

ISBN: 978-0-9961533-0-0

# Table of Contents

# Acknowledgments

We gratefully acknowledge the assistance and encouragement of our classmates at Duke and colleagues elsewhere. In particular, we are grateful for Allison Ta, Cristophe Hansen, Curry Cheek, Danielle Sobol, Emily Ngan, Jeff Smith, Jessica Friedman, Nathan Brajer, Rand Wilcox Vanden Berg, Rikesh Gandhi, Rui Dai, Sameer Hirji, and Toria Rendell, and Ryan Muller, whose generous feedback helped make the book you see today.

# Chapter 1:
## Introduction

As a medical student, learning is your job. But while med school does a fine job of transmitting knowledge, many schools do not teach students *how to learn*. That is what we wanted to change with this book.

This book is going to show you a new system for learning. We're going to teach you how to efficiently absorb and synthesize the material in your textbooks, even when the material seems impenetrable at first glance. We'll introduce software tools that will let you memorize anything and everything you need to, and retain it for the long haul. Finally, with these tools in place, we'll go through the major subjects you'll learn in med school, and show you how to put these principles into action, step by step.

What can you expect from these tools? First, they will help you excel on standardized tests such as the USMLE Step 1, which is used as an important criterion for acceptance into most residency programs. They will also help you perform well in school and on the wards, by effectively retaining as much knowledge as possible so that you can apply it on exams and during your patient care responsibilities. Most importantly, applying these lessons to learn more effectively will help you become a better doctor, better informed by your training, more able to stay on top of developments in your field. And also, by the same token, being more effective in your learning will free up time to connect with your patients and think more humanistically about the practice of medicine.

## At a Glance – What This Book Will Do For You

- Give you a basic understanding of how learning and memory work
- Provide you with powerful learning practices and the evidence that supports them
- Develop a complete learning methodology that you can apply throughout your career in medicine
- Help you to identify and employ useful digital tools for medicine
- Help you perform at a high level academically
- Equip you to become the best doctor you can be

# Our story

Alex and Peter, your humble co-authors, met as medical students at Duke. Alex is an MD/PhD student interested in pain medicine. Peter is an MD starting his training in radiology. Above all, we're passionate about medicine and effective learning.

Like most of you, when studying in college and prepping for the MCAT, we tried a number of different approaches – outlines, notecards, cramming, the works. But when we reached medical school, we were overwhelmed by the volume of information. We realized that these approaches weren't enough. Brute force would let us learn most of what we needed and pass the tests, but "good enough" wasn't enough for us.

Worse yet, with a pure cramming regimen, we'd start forgetting key concepts that we learned just a few weeks earlier. We heard well-meaning upperclassmen telling us "Don't worry – you'll forget it all by second year and you'll have to relearn it anyway." What a depressing thought! We needed to find a better strategy if we were going to learn and keep on top of all this information.

So we went to the literature on learning and memory, and sought out what science had to say about optimal ways to study. With some theory under our belts, we were better able to experiment and develop unconventional study strategies that far outperformed what we had been doing before. We talked with our classmates, who adopted parts of this methodology for themselves and offered useful suggestions to streamline it further.

It wasn't perfect. After all, it took years for us to learn how to study the old-fashioned way, and we were trying to implement a new one in just a few weeks. We made mistakes along the way, and as we kept talking to other students, we realized that many of them were running across similar stumbling blocks. We looked at the recurrent problems and figured out ways around them.

Pretty soon our class was teaching these techniques to the incoming first years, and a year later, that class started reaching out to the *new* incoming first years. And sure enough, many of us did very well on the USMLE step exams and found that we had a firm grasp of preclinical knowledge once we hit the wards – our studying yielded much better results than we could have otherwise expected.

We wrote this book because we wanted to both expand and improve on the methodology we've developed. We wanted to reach out to students beyond Duke to present them with a fully developed system so that they could hit the ground running in medical school and beyond. We wanted to write the book we wish had existed when we started our medical school journey.

# Who is this book for?

Our background is in medicine, and so we wrote this book with incoming first-year medical students in mind. We chose our examples and tailored our implementation to specifically help you navigate and get the absolute most out of medical school.

There's value here for grizzled med school veterans as well. If you're in your preclinical years, we can help you retain and systematize your learning in medical school. (We ourselves hadn't fleshed out our system completely until well into our preclinical education.) If you're on rotations, our system can help you make sense of the often haphazard clinical learning that comes at you on the wards. And for residents and beyond, lifelong learning is a way of life in medicine. As you deepen your knowledge of your specialty and stay abreast of the latest research, we want to equip you to be the best practitioner you can be.

That said, the principles we present are universal, and extend well beyond learning medicine. With a few tweaks you could use the same principles to learn any subject. Despite our title, we believe that the systematic approach to learning we advocate can be valuable for everyone. Other health professions students can find value here, adjusting implementation based on their own in-depth knowledge of how nursing school or physician assistant school is structured. Furthermore, what we're offering is a general, evidence-based approach to learning and retaining knowledge. And that's a tool that can help anyone, of any age, who approaches any body of knowledge as a student.

# How this book is organized

This book is organized to take the reader from theory to practice. The first section, *Brain Science*, explains the fundamental psychological principles of learning. Part II talks about spaced repetition software, the backbone of our learning method. It walks you through how to set up Anki, our preferred spaced repetition system, and explains how to use it to get the maximum benefit. Part III, *The Learning Method*, is a step-by-step description of how to study anything in medical school, whether from books, videos, or lectures. Part IV, *Implementation*, gives specific tips, tools, and frameworks to help you approach the diverse subjects you learn in medical school, from anatomy to pharmacology. Finally, in the final section, *The Future of Medicine*, we consider what skills a 21st century doctor might need beyond what's taught in medical school and suggest how you might teach yourself those skills.

# Our philosophy

When trying to decide how to learn, everyone comes at the problem with their own perspective, and we are no different. Since we in medicine believe in informed consent, let's lay out the three major principles that inform our approach in thinking about how to study for medical school.

## 1. Evidence-based learning

One dominant theme in modern medicine is the idea that the practice of medicine should be grounded in solid empirical evidence, whenever it is available. It even has a trendy name: "Evidence-Based Medicine" or EBM. You will hear this term throughout your medical career – and for good reason: if we want to achieve predictable and optimal outcomes, then we should look to the evidence to see what actually works. With something as serious as medicine, it sensible to insist on evidence-based methods.

But it also makes sense for any other endeavor in life where we want to achieve the best, most consistent results. As medical students, our job is to learn medicine, and we spend a tremendous amount of time, money and effort in doing that job. Shouldn't we strive to apply best practices to what we do? Shouldn't we make use of the available evidence about learning to guide our studies rather than just doing what seems right?

We certainly think so. Learning medicine is serious business, and it deserves to be treated that way. So we've gone to the literature on learning, memory, and psychology, and we've written the recommendations in this book based on the best available science. But there are still many things we don't know about learning and memory, especially in applying these findings to learning medicine. In those cases, we appeal to our experiences and those of other successful medical students. This, too, is analogous to the way doctors practice EBM. When solid evidence is lacking, they must integrate what they know with their expert experience and judgment.

## 2. Learning comes first

We all have our reasons for why we wanted to become doctors. Maybe we wanted to learn all about the amazing complexity of the human body. Maybe we wanted to do cutting-edge research to cure diseases. Or maybe we wanted a chance to show compassion and personally ease the suffering of our patients. Medicine can be all of these things, but it comes with something more – a deep responsibility for the well-being of our patients.

Let's run some numbers. Let's say you'll be practicing for 30 years – although many physicians practice well into their 70s and beyond. And let's give you a leisurely clinic schedule of 10 patients a day. This means that you'll have 75,000 patient visits over the course of your career. Many of them will be sniffles and scrapes – common problems that anyone with the right training can manage. But some of them will be more challenging, testing the limits of your diagnostic and management skills. This is where the depth of your knowledge will make a difference.

Let's say that one in 50 patients – 2% of them – have an unusual presentation or require unconventional treatment. They're the rare "zebras," the patients where you have to go above and beyond cookbook medicine. Over the course of your career, the number of such patients you will encounter is 1500. Let that sink in for a minute. Throughout medical school, residency, and the lifelong learning beyond, how well you learn your craft will determine whether these patients will get better or get worse. You will have a massive impact on 1500 lives.

That is why we aimed this book at helping you *learn* in medical school, rather than helping you *ace* medical school. Of course we want to help you succeed at all the steps along the way – med school grades, boards scores, and residency applications. And we think we can do a pretty good job. But at the end of the day, our responsibility is to our future patients, not to the testing agencies. Keeping an eye on this goal can help us stay focused on what's important, as well as motivate us and insulate us from burnout as we go through the challenges of medical school.

In this book, you'll see that we advocate some unconventional methods. We'll show you how to study in a new way. We'll encourage you to test out not going to lectures. We'll have you do additional reviews beyond what you need to ace your school exams. If we cared only about short-term goals – weekly quiz grades, giving the appearance of being a good student – these may not be the very best methods. But in our minds, helping to take better care of those 1500 patients is far more important than doing things by the book. If you apply our lessons, there's no reason you won't be very competitive, both in class and on the boards. But our ultimate goal, and hopefully your goal too, is to be the best doctor you can be. That's why we wrote this book. That's what we want to help you strive passionately towards.

# 3. Use of technology

Med school today looks a lot different than it did even a decade ago. In many schools, lectures are streamed online for students to watch at their own pace. New books and online resources have sprung up and become overnight classics. The computational power at our fingertips and in our pockets opens up entirely new ways of studying that were impossible in our professors' generations.

We're enthusiastic fans of using technology to augment our learning. We'll be practicing in a world where genomically targeted cancer therapy and robot-assisted surgery are commonplace. There's no reason that our studying should be any less high-tech. Books and lectures have an important place in our system, but we'll also be introducing you to online resources and computer-based tools that your professors may not be familiar with but that we think can supercharge your learning.

# Section I
## Brain Science

# Chapter 2:
# A Model Of The Mind

Over the past century, scientists have learned a great deal about how the mind works. Neuroscientists, cognitive psychologists, linguists, computer scientists and many others have expanded our understanding of the mind. In this section, we'll take a tour through our modern understanding of learning and memory, focusing on the key ideas that are necessary to discuss and understand our learning system.

Before coming to med school, neither of us thought much about the science of learning. But in our pursuit of finding the most effective methods for learning medicine, we were forced to do a deep dive into the literature of learning and memory, because only armed with this understanding could we identify the best ways to study and separate out fact from fiction.

> "Only armed with this understanding could we identify the best ways to study and separate out fact from fiction."

You're not looking to become neuroscientists. So why don't we just jump straight to our study strategies? Partly because we want you to understand the principles that underlie our recommendations. We've found that when people understand *why* something works, they are much more enthusiastic about it and more likely to stay committed. But also, we know that learning can never be one size fits all, and you'll want to modify our workflow to suit your goals. When you understand the basic principles on which our learning system is built, you'll be in a better position to take charge and create a study plan that best suits your needs.

This section is organized in two chapters. In the first, we will develop a simple model of the mind. In the second, we'll show how this model illuminates two important phenomena in effective learning, which will become the backbone of our learning methodology. By the end of these two chapters, we hope to show you that by using what we know about how learning works, we can better define those study strategies that get us outsized results. From there, we'll be well equipped to move on to how to apply these strategies to produce the most efficient study strategy possible.

# The Dual-Store model

You've probably heard the terms "short-term memory" and "long-term memory." We all have an intuition that memory comes in several forms, and that the goal of learning is to form durable memories that we can readily access later. But how does memory work, and how can we make it work better for us?

The **dual-store model** is an oversimplified yet useful yet useful model of the mind.[1] In this model, there are two distinct memory entities: working memory (short-term) and long-term memory. **Working memory** is a storage mechanism that holds information for a brief time, while **long-term memory** can hold information for much longer periods of time, on the order of hours to years.

The Dual-Store Model

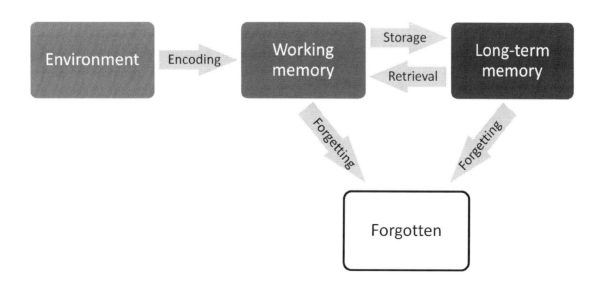

Information moves between the environment and these two types of memory through several processes. **Encoding** is the first step, where sensory input from the environment is changed into a form that the mind can store. For example, your eye sees photons of different frequencies and your mind transforms that raw sensory data into a mental image. **Storage** is the process of by which nascent memories are kept for later use. And finally, **retrieval** is the process by which memories are brought out of a long-term memory and sent to working memory so you can use it. The reverse of retrieval is **forgetting,** which is when material in long-term storage disappears or becomes inaccessible.[2]

In the following sections we'll take a closer look at the capabilities and weaknesses of each type of memory, and each of the processes that our brain uses to move information between them. You can guess that we'll be spending most of our effort trying to maximize encoding, storage, and retrieval while minimizing forgetting. But before we can figure out smart tactics for doing that, we need to understand more about how these forms of memory work in the first place.

## Environment and Attention

The **environment** provides all raw input for the mind. This includes all the sensory input coming in from all senses – the sounds of cars bustling down the street, the smell of a home cooked meal, the sight of a blue sky on a sunny day, and the feel of how your clothes hang on your body. This is a huge amount of information, and if we had no way to filter it down, we'd be overwhelmed. That's why our minds apply a filtering mechanism, **attention**, to allow only a fraction of raw sensory information to make it to our awareness.

## Working memory

Incoming information that makes it through the filter of attention then goes to a temporary holding area called **working memory**. Working memory is the part of the mind where our current thoughts reside, where we can ponder, calculate, and join thoughts together. Indeed, many brain scientists regard working memory as the seat of consciousness or thinking itself.[3]

But working memory is limited, both in capacity and in duration. Your conscious mind can only think about so many things at once. Researchers have tried to characterize the capacity of working memory for decades. The first and most famous estimate of how many items can reside in working memory at a given moment is Miller's "7 +/- 2" rule, which says that the average limit of working memory is 7 items, give or take.[3] More recent estimates put that number even lower, at four items.[4] The duration of working memory is also limited – to about 30 seconds.[5] Indeed, for this reason, working memory used to be called "short-term memory".[5]

These constraints of working memory have tremendous implications for learning. Indeed, cognitive scientist Daniel Willingham says "[the] lack of space in working memory is the fundamental bottleneck of human cognition." He goes on to say,

> You could dream up lots of ways that your cognitive system could be improved—more accurate memory, more focused attention, sharper vision, and so on—but if a genie comes out of a lamp and offers you one way to improve your mind, ask for more working memory capacity."[3]

Accordingly, many of the tactics we'll employ later on in the *Learning Method* section aim to circumvent these inherit limitations of working memory. So let's now discuss how we might do that.

## Chunking

No doubt you have been able to remember numbers longer than phone numbers, and perhaps even a credit card number, which has 16 digits or more. How is it that you can capture that and juggle it in your working memory?

The answer is that we must consider what the mind regards as an "item." In the case of the credit card numbers, you most likely grouped the digits into four blocks, reducing the total items in working memory to four. This is most obvious when we're thinking about words: your mind doesn't panic when it sees a word with more than four letters, but rather combines those letters together to make a meaningful word. By associating a meaning with the letters, you effectively compressed the information and reduced the cognitive burden on your working memory.

This process of information compression into meaningful units is called **chunking**, and it's a powerful strategy that the mind uses to overcome its own limits. When new information comes into working memory, we try very hard to make sense of that information, so as to compress the information and free up space for other items to enter the mental workspace.

Some of the study strategies we talk about later are helpful precisely by exploiting this capability. For example, in the *Implementation* section, we give you frameworks to help you think about each medical subject and break down the content into manageable chunks.

## Automaticity

Another way to get around the inherent limitations of working memory is make the access and application of basic knowledge automatic, without reflection. As you are reading this text, your mind is instantly processing the individual letters into words that convey meaning, without any conscious effort from you at all. Back in kindergarten, you laboriously and painstakingly looked at each letter to try to make out a simple word, but with much practice over the years, your mind just comprehends the words on this page automatically. Similarly, when you first started driving a car, it required conscious effort, but now you can hop in your car and wind up at your destination without even realizing all the maneuvers you made to get there. This is automaticity, and its purpose is to make key knowledge and skills so accessible that they don't need the cognitive resources of your working memory. This frees up more space to process new information and perform challenging mental tasks.

So how does one build automaticity? Practice and repetition. Cognitive scientist Daniel Willingham says it like this: "The development of automaticity for generalized skills depends on high levels of practice. There is no substitute."[6] Thus, to build automaticity to overcome the limits of working memory, we must do something over and over. In the next chapter, we'll discuss specific ways to practice that will help you to make your learning automatic.

## Long-term memory

In addition to working memory, the mind also has **long-term memory,** which is a vast repository of factual and procedural knowledge. Unlike working memory, its capacity is nearly limitless, and the memories that reside here have variable durations, from several hours to years to entire lifetimes. The goal of medical school, of course, is for your knowledge to end up here: stored securely, available to be transferred to working memory when we need it.

Unlike working memory, though, the storehouse of long-term memory remains mostly out of consciousness. We can't be aware of all its contents at once. Rather, when we want to access certain memories from this storehouse, we must retrieve them and bring them into working memory. If we want to have knowledge at our fingertips, we also have to focus on the process of retrieval.

Now that we've described the major components of the mind, let's discuss the processes that move information between each of these components: learning, retrieval, and forgetting.

# Learning

We've described how information comes in from the environment, gets filtered by attention, and makes its way to working memory. But what happens to that new information? There are two possible fates. The information either gets forgotten, or it is sent for archiving in long-term memory; this is what we refer to as **learning**.

When it comes to learning, all information is not created equal. If this weren't the case, we'd remember a random grab-bag of information throughout our lives. We'd be as likely to remember the multiplication table as we would be to remember what shirt we wore on a random day in first grade. In fact, how likely we are to learn something depends on several variables, including our ability to find meaning in it, how we organize it and the sensory modalities we use to process it. Let's explore each of these factors and see how we can make use of them in our studies.

# Meaningful learning

A key insight from the learning and memory literature is that meaningful information is more effectively stored than meaningless information.[3] Let's compare two pieces of information, both 14 characters long:

A. 47484294842716

B. TET3 is a protein

If I were to ask you to recall these items a week from now, which do you think you would be more likely to remember? No doubt (B). Why is "TET3 is a protein" so much easier to remember than the random number in (A)?

The answer is that the second sentence has meaning for you. You may not have ever heard of TET3 before, but you most certainly know what a protein is. You can connect TET3 with all the past knowledge you have about proteins (i.e. that they are made of amino acids, they have distinct biological functions, etc.). The memories you have of 'proteins' serve as an anchor for the new knowledge about TET3, which you can use in the future to try to remember it. On the other hand, (A) has no meaning for you, other than that you know what numbers are. That's what makes it so hard to remember. Learning information that has meaning is much easier than learning random facts. Meaningful learning is more powerful than rote learning.[1]

A corollary is that in order to take advantage of meaningful learning, we need to have preexisting knowledge to connect to new information. So, if we want to learn about a subject that is new to us, we can't dive right in and try to know every detail. On the contrary, it's better to ease in, approaching the landscape from a high level. Then, when we've gotten enough of an overview to have a foundation, we can go deeper. In our learning method, we call this the "three view model" We recommend making three passes at new knowledge, going from a high level overview to a nitty-gritty detailed view at the end.

> "To take advantage of meaningful learning, we need to have preexisting knowledge to connect to new information."

## Organization aids memory

The process of retrieval is like searching through a vast warehouse of memories and trying to find the right one, a veritable needle in the haystack kind of task. A well-organized warehouse is easier to search through than one that is a mess. So too with our memory. Organizing knowledge makes it easier to find things later.

For example, when you learn physical exam techniques, it's common to organize those techniques anatomically, going from head to toe. In this case, you use the inherent spatial properties of the human body to group certain pieces of knowledge. When you then perform the exam in the clinic, you don't just try to remember all techniques at once; instead, you use the anatomical organization to guide you along, first doing the head and neck, then moving to the thoracic region and beyond.

Categorization is another common way to organize information. Indeed, categorizing things is so natural to us that we do it automatically. For example, if we're learning about pathology of the heart, we can group different diseases by their shared properties. Mitral stenosis, mitral proplapse and aortic stenosis are categorized as "valvular diseases" while myocardial infarction would fall under the heading of 'ischemic disease'. Using groupings like this to arrange related pieces of knowledge is very useful, as it allows us to find these memories in predictable places.

Mental models that represent cause-effect relationships are also an important and effective way to organize knowledge. Let's consider the renin-angiotensin system, which is the body's way of homeostatically regulating blood pressure. Medical students are commonly asked to use use this knowledge is to predict and explain the body's response to decreased blood volume. The linear causal model of this response would look like this:

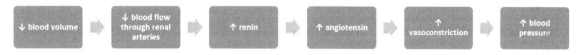

Each one of the components of this model means little on its own. But when strung together in sequence, important relationships emerge. Moreover, when you go to recall it, your recall of one component triggers the next. You don't need to call up all these ideas into your conscious mind (working memory) all at once. Rather, you can think about one pair at a time, and the previous item (lower blood volume) triggers the next (less blood flow). In this way, the mind eventually works its way to the final response in a reliable, memorable way. The organization of this causal model makes retrieval more reliable, and also provides much more useful and predictive information, since ideas and relationships are contained in it.

## Visual imagery

Finally, the mind finds it easier to remember information that leverages visual imagery rather than those that don't.[22] Consider two lists of words:

(1) – tree, apple, cigarette
(2) – love, happiness, fear

If you were asked to remember these lists and recall them tomorrow, which do you suspect would be easier to recall? If you picked list (1), then you'd be right. The reason is that these words are concrete words that have strong visual images associated with them, as opposed to list (2) which are all abstract words. To learn the concrete list, your mind forms connections to both the meaning of the words *and* their images, while it can only work with the meanings of the abstract list.

Practically speaking, you can enhance learning by tying new information with strong mental pictures. **Mnemonics**, which are common learning devices, very often use vivid imagery to help people remember information. The classic mnemonic for the cranial nerves paints a rather silly, but memorable, picture: "On Old Olympus's Tower Top, A Finn And German Viewed Some Hops." Taking it to the next level, many memory

> "You can enhance learning by tying new information with strong mental pictures."

champions use **memory palaces** to make connections between facts they're learning and a visualized room, to strengthen their memory by exploiting the visual and spatial orientation of their memory palace.

Indeed, several resources for learning medicine make heavy use of visual imagery. These include platforms like Picmonic, SketchyMicro and the textbook, *Clinical Microbiology Made Ridiculously Simple*. The popularity of these tools is a testament to the power of using images to learn complex information.

## Retrieval

The memories that reside in long-term memory are out of awareness. Only when we access them and move them into working memory do they come into our conscious awareness and can then be manipulated and combined in new ways. This process of pulling memories from the long-term storage into working memory is called **retrieval**.

Being able to reliably and rapidly perform retrieval is the purpose of learning. After all, if something resides in your long-term memory but you can't retrieve it, it's as good as gone. Fortunately, there are some ways to structure your learning to enhance retrieval later.

## On Context and Process

Memories are associated with contexts. The aroma of chocolate chip cookies may bring you back to a moment from your childhood, sitting in grandma's kitchen on a summer afternoon. Or a specific fragrance, maybe a cologne or perfume, may take you back to a very exact moment in your past, such as your first date in high school. In these cases, your mind associated those smells with your environmental context, and smelling the odor again is a trigger for your mind to find a memory.

Factual knowledge works the same way. Learning is most effective when the context at the time of learning matches the context at the time of retrieval, a principle called **encoding specificity**. Learning during the clinical year highlights how encoding specificity works. Let's say you're in the OR helping out on an appendectomy, and your attending tells you that appendicitis is most common between the ages of 5 to 40. Later that week, you're on the floor, and your resident pimps you about the demographics of appendicitis. You remember your attending just told you the other day, but try as you do, you can't remember. Your resident makes a sad face and doesn't tell you the answer. But then, you're in the OR again, and you're doing another appendicitis. Your resident asks you again, and this time, you rattle off "between the age of 5 and 40" like a champ. How the heck did that happen? You didn't know it on the floor, but you do in the OR. What is happening here? It's about context. Being in the OR again, with its distinctive sounds, sights and smells, as well as your emotional state from being barked at by a surgeon, helped you to recreate the original context where you first learned this factoid. The context helped your mind trace back easily to the memory in a way you couldn't on the floor, where the contextual cues were missing.

A related principle, **transfer-appropriate processing (TAP),** suggests that you should learn something in the same way that you plan to use it later on, to take advantage of process similarities. For example, if you're learning how to do ACLS (a form of CPR), and you know that you will be later tested in a real simulation environment where you'll need to physically perform ACLS procedures on a dummy, then TAP would argue that you should learn and practice ACLS in the same way – physically going through the steps, in as realistic an environment as possible. Spending many hours reading about ACLS and watching videos, although beneficial, would not work as well, since in this type of

> "You should learn something in the same way that you plan to use it later on,"

learning you're engaging different processes (watching and hearing) than you would in the real test situation. We can sum up the guidance here as "practice how you'll perform".

## Retrieval begets more retrieval

Research has shown that one of the most powerful ways to enhance retrieval is to do more of it.[7-9] Retrieving begets more and better retrieval in the future. Thus, if you want to remember something long-term, the best course of action to is practice retrieval of that piece of information. This idea is called the **testing effect**. We introduce this idea here just for completeness, but there is much more to say. We will dedicate the entire next chapter to exploring the power of the testing effect.

## Forgetting

We can't talk about memory without talk about **forgetting,** which is a failure to re-member. Forgetting erodes our learning, thus we want to minimize it as best we can. To do that, we must understand a bit more about what forgetting is and how it happens.

You might think that forgetting is about erasure of old memories. But many neuro-scientists have increasingly looked at forgetting as a *failure in retrieval* of a memory. In this view, it's not so much about not having the memory in our long-term storage, but rather an inability to find and retrieve a memory from storage. So in future chapters, we'll focus on ways to build and strengthen retrieval as an important ingredient in combatting forgetting.

# Bring It All Together – A summary of the Dual-Store model

Before we move on, let's have another look at the dual-store model and review what we've learned.

Input from the environment (information) is encoded and enters into working memory in a process strongly determined by what we choose to focus our attention on. The lifetime of these new short-term memories is ephemeral. You have to do something to move memories from here into long-term storage. We have some tricks, such as chunking and repetition, extending the capacity and lifetime of working memory a little bit, but in order to really move on to the long-term storage, information in working memory must undergo effortful processing. Some strategies toward that end are meaningful learning, organization and visual imagery. Memories in long-term memory are normally out of conscious awareness, but when certain information is needed, these memories can be retrieved and brought back into working memory. Finally, if nothing is done to preserve them, long-term memories can decay by forgetting.

In this chapter, we've focused mostly on techniques that aid in the uptake of new information, but in the next chapter, we'll introduce two very potent tools that aid on the recall side, namely **spaced practice** and **retrieval practice.** These two methods are so effective that we've made them the backbone of our learning system.

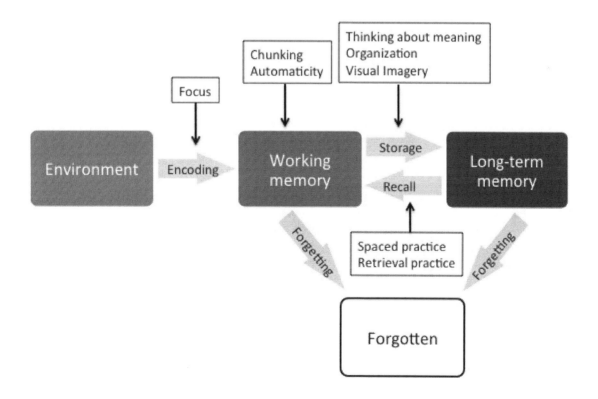

# Chapter 3:
# Spacing And Testing – The Best Study Strategies You Never Heard Of

With our model of memory, we can now turn our attention to two key observations about how people learn: the **spacing effect** and the **testing effect**. The spacing effect tells us how to schedule our studying to maximize learning; the testing effect shows us how to study to minimize forgetting. These phenomena are some of the most reliable and robust findings in all of cognitive psychology. Because of their power, we've made **spaced repetition**, a technique that exploits these effects, the backbone of our learning system. We'll talk more about how spaced repetition works in the next chapter. In this chapter, however, we'll go into detail about the spacing and testing effects and their implications for learning.

## The Forgetting Curve and the Spacing Effect

More than 100 years ago, a German psychologist named Hermann Ebbinghaus made one of the most critical discoveries about memory. Ebbinghaus had performed numerous experiments testing his own memory using lists of nonsense syllables. He would read the lists out loud and then immediately try to recall them correctly. If he could not recall correctly, he would re-read the lists and then try again until he could get it right.

From these experiments, Ebbinghaus made several remarkable discoveries. First, he found that forgetting followed a predictable pattern. Below you can see a graph (adapted from the original) of Ebbinghaus' seminal finding about the relationship between memory and retention interval. Just after learning some new material, within the first hour or so, retention is very high. But shortly after, within the first 24 hours, retention falls very rapidly to less than 40% and then levels off in subsequent days. This representation of forgetting is aptly called the **Forgetting Curve**. The takeaway is as clear as it is discouraging: we forget a lot and we forget very quickly. In light of the Forgetting Curve, it's almost a wonder that we remember anything at all.

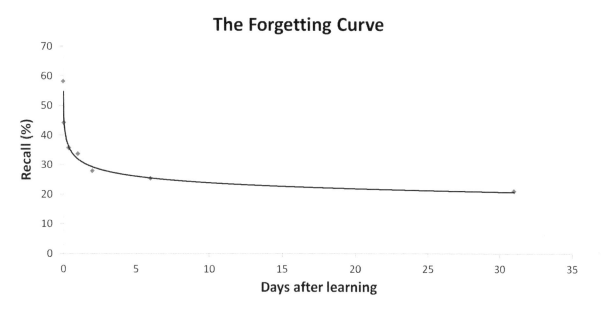

Thankfully, another of Ebbinghaus' findings is the silver lining to this dark cloud. Ebbinghaus found that practicing can slow down forgetting. And the more times he repeated learning his lists on day 1, the less time he would need to spend re-learning in subsequent days. The message is that forgetting can be thwarted by repeated practice.

Ebbinghaus made another key observation: *when* you study matters more than *how often* you study. In one of his experiments, Ebbinghaus arranged his studying efforts in two ways. In one case, he crammed 68 successive reviews and then tested himself the next day to see how much he could remember. He then took the same material and spaced out his learning over the course of three days, but only doing 38 repetitions. At the end of those three days, he tested himself to see how much he could remember. Here's Ebbinghaus describing the results:

"38 repetitions, distributed in a certain way over the three preceding days, **has just as favorable an effect as 68 repetitions made on the day just previous** … This makes the assumption probable that with any considerable number of repetitions a suitable distribution of them over a space of time is decidedly more advantageous than the massing of them at a single time."[23]

Ebbinghaus got the same results with nearly half the effort when he spaced out this learning rather than cramming.

These results gave rise to what has been called the **spacing effect**: "learning events that are repeated over time result in more efficient learning and greater retention compared to exposure to a single bolus of material."[10] The spacing effect has been studied and validated many times since Ebbinghaus first

*"Ebbinghaus got the same results with nearly half the effort when he spaced out this learning rather than cramming."*

described it. Indeed, according to one recent article, "the spacing effect is arguably the most replicable and robust finding from experimental psychology. Hundreds of articles,

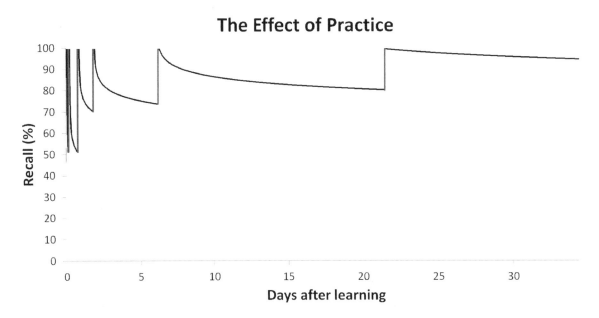

**The Effect of Practice**

Recall (%) vs. Days after learning

Adapted from Wolf G. "Want to Remember Everything You'll Ever Learn? Surrender to This Algorithm" Wired. (2008)

including a number of reviews and meta-analyses, have found a spacing effect in a wide variety of memory tasks."[11]

Some of these studies further refined the spacing schedules, and the required number of repetitions fell still lower. Using the Forgetting Curve and our knowledge of the decay rate of knowledge, we can create algorithms to predict, with uncanny accuracy, just when we're most likely to forget a fact. By timing our study sessions appropriately, we can significantly extend our memory.

# The Spacing Effect in action

In one study, two groups of students were taught how to do a particular kind of math problem, one with spacing and the other with massed practice, which is the repeated presentation of to-be-learned material in a short period of time (i.e. cramming). Although both groups did similarly on a test one week after studying, the spacing group scored almost *double* the massed practice group on the test for weeks afterwards. Similar effects were found in eighth-graders learning about US history, as well as first-graders learning how to read.[12]

Studies focusing on medical education are more limited, but still show support for the value of spacing in medical school. In one randomized controlled trial, Kerfoot *et al.* looked at the impact of the spacing effect on retention of physical exam skills among medical students at Harvard. All the students received clinical teaching about how to perform physical exams. Then, one group got a set of questions emailed to them once a week for three weeks, while the other group only got one week of emails. At the end of the course, the group that had three cycles of emails scored 74% correctly on the exam, compared to 59% for students who only got one cycle of email. Despite the minor time obligation to complete the emailed questions, 85% of participants recommended the spacing program for the next year's class. This study shows that spaced repetition can work well for medical school, even on the relatively short time scales of a physical exam course.[13] We can expect the benefits of spacing to only increase as time goes on.

Recently, the effectiveness of spaced learning has been extended from the medical undergraduate level up to practicing primary care physicians. In a randomized study, Kerfoot *et al.* demonstrated that use of an online spaced education game can help physicians more effectively achieve blood pressure control in hypertensive patients.[14] This note-worthy finding demonstrates that the benefits of spaced repetition extend not only to the learners themselves, but also to their patients.

# Cramming: A Faustian bargain

You may have noticed something funny here. From what we're saying, it seems that the spacing effect can help us retain more while studying less. Yet many of us have gotten quite far in our academic careers by doing exactly the opposite, through intensive cramming just before an exam. If cramming is so inefficient, then why does everyone do it?

Cramming *does* work well in the short term. There is no denying that. You can load up your memory with information and some of it will stay there for a time. But as anyone who has ever crammed for a test can confirm, the gains are merely temporary. This is often good enough to pass weekly quizzes, and do well on tests without strongly cumulative elements. And since many classes are set up that way, cramming is often one way to get a good grade. But at the end of the day, all those efforts produce very little long-term knowledge.

Think about all that time and money you spent in college trying to learn for classes. How much of it do you remember now? The same goes for med school, with even more troubling consequences. A standard piece of advice for incoming medical students is "don't get overwhelmed by coursework, you'll have to re-learn it later anyway." This advice takes for granted that we're cramming, and that our knowledge from each course is going to rapidly decay. Well, in that case, how much will be left when we're seeing patients?

Too often, medical school curricula promote cramming with their reliance on short term tasks and examinations. So we cram and then move on. This transforms medical school into what we call "academic theater": it gives the appearance that everybody has learned the material well, but in fact, if you come back a week later, you'll find that few could recall most of what they've "learned."

Because of this arrangement, the temptation to cram is always going to be there. The goal of our learning system is to break this cycle and help you build durable, life-long knowledge. The spacing effect is a key component in that effort.

# The Testing Effect – Testing's not just for exams anymore

In 1918, Arthur Gates published a study in which grade school students in Oakland, California were given two items to learn: a set of nonsense syllables and a paragraph containing a brief biography. One set was told to study by reading the study materials from beginning to end until the time was up. The other half was told to quiz themselves by trying to reproduce the syllables and biography, then to check their memory against their study materials. They were then quizzed twice, once after eight minutes to assess learning, and then again 3 to 4 hours later to test for retention. In every case, and within each grade, the students that spent more time quizzing themselves performed decisively better than those who passively read their study materials. The effects were particularly pronounced on the retention test, where self quizzers had around a 50% advantage for the biographical materials and almost a *fourfold advantage* in learning nonsense syllables.[15]

Gates' finding that quizzing yourself results in better recall has been observed in many more settings since, giving rise to the phenomenon known as the **testing effect**. The testing effect is the finding that testing produces superior long-term retention compared to passive review. If you're going to study, you're much better off asking yourself questions about what you're trying to learn rather than passively rereading your notes or textbook.

Keep in mind that the word *testing* in this context doesn't refer to formal examinations in school. Rather, it is a more general term equivalent to retrieval; that is, trying to pull out a memory from long-term memory.

If we think about it, the testing effect is a specific application of the principles of the

> "Testing produces superior long-term retention compared to passive review."

dual-store model we introduced last chapter. Testing forces you to practice retrieval. Each time you test yourself, your mind reorganizes the way it stores the information, and generates clearer pathways to retrieve knowledge. Ultimately, this both strengthens your retrieval, and reduces the mental burden to recall a fact, which also helps to decrease the demand on your working memory. Retrieval becomes automatic, and you have the fact ready at hand whenever you need it.

# The Spacing and Testing Effects in action

Some recent studies have really brought the testing effect to the forefront. We'll take a look at a few of these studies – some on learning in general, some explicitly about medical education – to give you a sense of the exciting research backing up the spacing and testing effects.

An important study by Blunt *et al.* in the journal *Science* compared two learning strategies: testing and concept-mapping.[16] They chose to make the comparison to concept-mapping because it's seen as one of the most effective most effective learning strategies by educators, since it's active and requires thought, not just passive review. The researchers divided 80 undergraduates into four different groups and had all the subjects from each group read a biology text. One group did no further studying after the initial reading ("study once" group). Another group was instructed to read the text four more times consecutively ("cramming" group). The third group read the text initially and then created a concept map corresponding to the text ("concept mapping" group). Lastly, in the "testing" group, the students read the text initially, and then did a free recall of anything they could remember from the reading. They then read the text again and did a free recall after that second reading. Importantly, the total time studying in the testing group was no different than that in the concept mapping groups; it's not as though they simply spent more time studying.

One week later, all four groups were called back to take a final short answer test on the passage they had read. This test addressed both verbatim questions and inferential questions that went beyond what was stated in the reading. The results were dramatic. The study once group got less than 30% correct, on average. The repeated study group did slightly better at 45% correct. The concept mapping group scored 40% correct. And the testing group? They got more than 60% correct on the test. In other words, the testing group experienced a 50% relative increase in recall performance when compared to the concept mapping group, all for the same amount of study time!

> "In other words, the testing group experienced a 50% relative increase in recall performance"

In a second experiment, which used a crossover design, the study authors instructed each individual student to read the same two texts, using retrieval practice (testing) for one text and concept mapping for another. A week later, subjects were called back for a final test that addressed the material from both texts. Half the subjects took a final short answer test and the other half took a final concept mapping test.

As in the first experiment, the subjects who repeatedly tested themselves (retrieval practice) initially achieved a significantly higher proportion correct on the short-answer test. But the especially interesting result was that **subjects who used studied using retrieval practice performed better on the final concept mapping test than the students who studied using concept mapping.** They beat them at their own game! The key takeaway from this study is any *individual* student can see benefits from switching to retrieval practice. How you study matters, irrespective of your innate intelligence or abilities.

# Testing in medicine

What about medicine? Here too there is increasing evidence that testing, also known as retrieval practice, can have substantial impact on long-term retention of biomedical knowledge.

One study by Schmidmaier *et al.* looked at a group of German medical students learning about nephrology, using electronic flashcards based on the popular CASUS™ learning system. Half of the students reviewed material by testing themselves; the other half reviewed by restudying the material. One week out, the testing group achieved 40% recall compared to 27% recall with restudying. However, at 6 months, both testing and restudying showed only 11% recall. While these findings do support the superior efficacy of testing, at the same time, it's clear that one study session really wasn't enough. As we learned from the spacing effect, long-term retention requires continued retrieval practice over time. With additional study sessions with carefully calibrated spacing intervals, we can do significantly better than the students in this study. We'll talk more about how to implement that in the next chapter.

Another study by Larsen *et al.* corroborated the usefulness of testing with a crossover study involving pediatric and emergency medicine residents.[17] In this study, the subjects attended a didactic conference that addressed myasthenia gravis (MG) and status epilepticus (SE). The subjects were randomized into two groups. One group was assigned to do repeated testing on status epilepticus but repeated study (with a standard review sheet) on myasthenia gravis. The other group did the opposite, testing repeatedly on myasthenia gravis but studying repeatedly on status epilepticus. After the initial teaching session, the subjects took the tests and did their studying during a timed block. Every two weeks for a month, they were called back to study the material (via both testing and passive review.)

On the initial test that followed the didactic conference, the residents scored fairly high on both SE (78%) and MG (62%). At the second testing, those scores dropped to 47% for SE and 44% for MG, and at the third testing, they came back up slightly to 55% for SE and 48% for MG.

But here is the most interesting part. At 6 months – after 5 months of no reviews or testing – the subjects were called back for a final test. For SE, the group that repeatedly tested on SE scored 42% on questions for SE, compared to 31% for the repeated study group, an 11% difference. The same thing was found on the MG side: the repeated testing group scored 36% correct while the repeated study group scored a mere 19% correct, a 17% difference.

The major conclusion is that repeated testing produces superior long-term retention of medical knowledge compared to repeated studying.

But we should put that conclusion into context. Over the course of six months, the residents lost a ton of knowledge. Testing helped attenuate the loss, but our take-away should be that whenever we learn something new, we quickly begin to forget it. If we don't do anything, this is the default: most of our hard-won knowledge will be lost. Testing was helpful in retaining some knowledge, but, as in the Schmidmaier study, there is significant room for improvement from optimizing the spacing interval.

> "The major conclusion is that repeated testing produces superior long-term retention of medical knowledge over repeated studying."

Just as with spacing, the testing effect holds true beyond the medical undergraduate level, as demonstrated by another recent study by Larsen *et al.*[18] In this study, physicians who attended a continuing medical education (CME) conference in neurology were instructed to either repeatedly quiz or repeatedly study material relevant to the conference. More than 5 months later, the same physicians were given a final test to assess their long-term retention of the knowledge they'd gained from the CME conference. Not surprisingly, repeated testing was superior, with physicians from this group reaching 55% correct on the final test vs. 44% in the repeated study group. Taken together, it is clear that retrieval practice (or testing) is a highly effective strategy for building durable knowledge across the physician's lifespan, from medical student to practicing physician.

# The Testing Effect and Skill Acquisition

While much of the literature on the testing effect in medicine has focused on retention of factual knowledge, clinical medicine also involves a great deal of skill-learning, and several other studies have shown that the testing effect works for skill learning just like it does for book learning.

Kromann *et al.* assessed the impact of the testing effect on learning resuscitation skills.[19] These are literally life-saving skills and have been shown to decay rapidly after an initial training course. The subjects for this study – medical students – took a short course on resuscitation skills. After the course, subjects either participated in a simulated cardiac arrest scenario (test) or reviewed several resuscitation scenarios with an instructor (control). Two weeks later, the subjects were called back and were assessed using a cardiac arrest scenario different from the ones that were used for training. The 'test' group had a mean score of 82.8% on the final assessment while the 'control' group had a mean score of 73.3%, demonstrating again the superiority of testing compared to other methods, even with just a single instance of testing.

Similar results were found by Kerfoot *et al.* in a large study of urology residents. This study found that repeated testing on questions of histopathological diagnosis produced superior long term retention compared to repeated web-based teaching modules. Repeated testing produced a mean long-term score increase in of 15.2% while repeated teaching produced a mere 3.4% score increase.[20]

# Metacognition in learning: You can't handle the truth!

You'd think that if testing were so obviously superior, everyone would know this and use it for their own studying. Similarly, you'd think that if the truth about the cost of cramming came out, people would stop cramming.

However, in a followup to their study comparing testing to concept mapping, Blunt *et al.* demonstrated that students don't always know what methods are effective, even when they try out and compare different study tactics.

Recall that the study by Blunt *et al.* compared concept mapping to testing, and found that testing was superior. But before they showed them the results, the authors asked students whether they thought retrieval practice or concept mapping would give them the best results. Overall, students predicted that repeated study (reading and re-reading) would be the best, followed by concept mapping, then retrieval, and finally study-once. Strange! Even after trying several approaches, *and* taking the exams that tested their knowledge, their intuition about what works was exactly the reverse of the truth! Indeed, in a prior study, Karpicke *et al.* remarked:

> "Students generally exhibit little awareness of the fact that practising retrieval enhances learning… When students rely purely on their subjective experience while they study (e.g., their fluency of processing during rereading) they may fall prey to illusions of competence and believe they know the material better than they actually do."[21]

We've seen this pattern firsthand in medical school, where people will work very hard using suboptimal methods, like repeated study, when superior methods are available to them. Intuition isn't good enough to determine what strategies actually help you learn. That's why we advocate going straight to the best literature on best practices rather than just going with your gut.

*"Students don't always know what methods are effective, even when they try out and compare different study tactics."*

# From theory to practice

This concludes our exploration of the literature on learning. We've talked about how the brain treats working memory as well as long-term memory, and the processes that lead to learning, retrieval, and forgetting. We've also explored some of the evidence for two key study strategies, spacing and testing, that have an outsized effect on learning and retention. We've gone into some detail on the studies demonstrating that these principles hold over a wide range of applications, especially in medicine.

From here, we move onwards from theory to practice. How do we integrate these principles efficiently into our study habits, without adding additional burdens on our already strained schedules? That will be the topic of the next sections of this book.

# References for Section I – Brain Science

1. Ormrod, J. E. *Human Learning*. (Pearson, 2012).

2. McLeod, S. Memory, Encoding Storage and Retrieval | Simply Psychology. (2007). at <http://www.simplypsychology.org/memory.html>

3. Willingham, D. T. *Why don't students like school: A cognitive scientist answers questions about how the mind works and what it means for the classroom.* (2009).

4. Lieberman, D. A. *Human Learning and Memory*. (Cambridge University Press, 2012).

5. Reisberg, D. *Cognition*. (W.W. Norton, 2010).

6. Willingham, D. T. Ask the Cognitive Scientist.

7. Dunlosky, J., Rawson, K.A., Marsh, E.J., Nathan, M.J., and Willingham, D.T. (2013). Improving students' learning with effective learning techniques promising directions from cognitive and educational psychology. *Psychological Science in the Public Interest* 14, 4–58.

8. Dunn, D. S., Saville, B. K. & Baker, S. C. Evidence-based teaching: Tools and techniques that promote learning in the psychology classroom. *Australian Journal of Psychology* 65, 5–13 (2013).

9. Karpicke, J. D. & Grimaldi, P. J. Retrieval-based learning: A perspective for enhancing meaningful learning. *Educational Psychology Review* 1–18 (2012).

10. Stahl, S. M. *et al.* Play it Again: The Master Psychopharmacology Program as an Example of Interval Learning in Bite-Sized Portions. *CNS Spectr* **15,** (2010).

11. Vlach, H. A. & Sandhofer, C. M. Distributing learning over time: The spacing effect in children's acquisition and generalization of science concepts. *Child development* 83, 1137–1144 (2012).

12. Carpenter, S. K., Cepeda, N. J., Rohrer, D., Kang, S. H. K. & Pashler, H. Using spacing to enhance diverse forms of learning: Review of recent research and implications for instruction. *Educational Psychology Review* 1–10 (2012). doi:10.1007/s10648-012-9205-z

13. Kerfoot, B. P., Armstrong, E. G. & O'Sullivan, P. N. Interactive spaced-education to teach the physical examination: a randomized controlled trial. *J Gen Intern Med* 23, 973–978 (2008).

14. Kerfoot, B. P., Turchin, A., Breydo, E., Gagnon, D. & Conlin, P. R. An online spaced-education game among clinicians improves their pat… - PubMed - NCBI. *Circulation: Cardiovascular Quality and Outcomes* 7, 468–474 (2014).

15. Gates, A. I. Correlations of immediate and delayed recall. *Journal of Educational Psychology* **9,** 489–496 (1918).

16. Karpicke, J. D. & Blunt, J. R. Retrieval Practice Produces More Learning than Elaborative Studying with Concept Mapping. *Science* **331,** 772–775 (2011).

17. Larsen, D.P., Butler, A.C., and Roediger, H.L., III (2009). Repeated testing improves long-term retention relative to repeated study: a randomised controlled trial. *Medical Education* 43, 1174–1181.

18. Larsen, D.P., Butler, A.C., Aung, W.Y., Corboy, J.R., Friedman, D.I., and Sperling, M.R. (2015). The effects of test-enhanced learning on long-term retention in AAN annual meeting courses. *Neurology* 84, 748–754.

19. Kromann, C.B., Jensen, M.L., and Ringsted, C. (2009). The effect of testing on skills learning. Medical Education 43, 21–27.

20. Kerfoot, B.P., Fu, Y., Baker, H., Connelly, D., Ritchey, M.L., and Genega, E.M. (2010). Online spaced education generates transfer and improves long-term retention of diagnostic skills: a randomized controlled trial. *J. Am. Coll. Surg.* 211, 331–337.e331.

21. Karpicke, J. D., Butler, A. C. & Roediger, H. L., III. Metacognitive strategies in student learning: Do students practise retrieval when they study on their own? *Memory* **17,** 471–479 (2009).

22. Medina, J. (2008). *Brain rules: 12 principles for surviving and thriving at work, home, and school.* Seattle: Pear Press.

23: Ebbinghaus, H. (1885) *Memory: A Contribution to Experimental Psychology*

# Section II
## Your Peripheral Brain: Spaced Repetition Software and Personal Notes

# Chapter 4:
# Spaced Repetition Apps – Supercharging Your Memory

Now that we know a little bit about the science of learning, how are we going to apply it? One obvious way is to apply the spacing and testing effects to enhance our memory, letting us retain much more of what we learn. We've discussed some straightforward ways to apply these principles. One way to take advantage of the testing effect would be to ask yourself questions while you study. Likewise, you could exploit the spacing effect by scheduling spreading your reviews out over time.

But using the spacing effect is harder than it looks. After all, not all facts are created equal. Some are easy to remember (the brain has four lobes) and some are hard (quick: draw the citric acid cycle!) You would want to use spaced repetition on both facts, but you'd want to review the citric acid cycle more often. Extend this throughout the entirety of med school, and you'll need to come up with a schedule for thousands of facts – a seemingly impossible task. But this is the age of computers, and we now have technology that makes efficient and effective studying much easier.

This technology is called spaced repetition software (SRS). There are several SRS apps available, which we'll discuss later. But at their core, SRS apps have the same central function: to enable you to review information repeatedly in a spaced manner. Most SRS apps use a kind flashcard interface, with a question or prompt on one side, and the answer on the other side. After you provide an answer, you must indicate whether it was correct or incorrect. Some SRS programs go a step further and have you provide a rating of how easily you recalled the information as well.

Using your performance data, SRS apps then manage when you should see that piece of information again in the future. This is where the available SRS apps diverge. Some SRS apps use a fixed time schedule while others using expanding interval scheduling.

Fixed scheduling presents reviews at constant intervals, e.g. every 3 days. In contrast, SRS apps that use an expanding interval schedule will present information after increasingly long delays. For example, if you answer a question correctly the first time you see it, you will see it again fairly soon, say one day later. But then, when you see that card and answer correctly again, the time until the next review will be further into the future, perhaps 3 days. Each time you answer a card correctly, the interval gets longer, on the order of months and years. In contrast, if you answer a card incorrectly, that's an indication that you need to see review that information soon, perhaps in a few hours. After you get it right, then the intervals will expand.

"SRS gives you the spacing and testing effects for free – without ever having to keep track of what fact to study when."

In addition, the scheduling time can also be modulated by the ease of recall. SRS programs such as Anki, Supermemo, and Firecracker use difficulty rating to adjust the future review schedule. Cards marked as easy get spaced farther apart than cards marked as hard.

Although there are many flavors of SRS, the bottom line is SRS programs are powerful tools for knowledge retention. SRS gives you the spacing and testing effects for free – without ever having to keep track of what fact to study when.

It's the engine for our entire learning strategy. It has so many benefits, we think it's important to elaborate them here.

## The Power of Spaced Repetition Software

That Spaced Repetition Software is effective should not be surprising, since it takes advantage of the robust and reproducible cognitive phenomena we discussed in the previous chapter. But you don't have to take our word for it.

Spaced repetition software has helped people achieve tremendous success in learning. One amazing example is that of Jeopardy contestant Roger Craig. Craig holds the record for highest single-day total of money ever won on Jeopardy, as well as the highest 5 day total. Craig, a computer scientist, used Anki, a popular, open-source SRS (more on Anki later), to help him remember facts he thought would show up in the game. His success is a testament to the efficacy of SRS.

How about SRS in medicine? Here, the evicence is inevitably anecdotal. Our personal experience – and those of many of our classmates who've used it – is that it helped us perform much better on the wards and on board exams than we would have otherwise. Our personal performance statistics in Anki, which is the SRS that we both used, demonstrate that we've gotten about 85-90% correct. Looking back at our medical school career, these statistics also reveal a steady pattern of increasing accuracy over time. That means that over the course of 2 years, we've been able to recall the vast majority of reviews – for over tens of thousands of medical facts. Our classmates who have tried Anki along with us, and the underclassmen who've taken up Anki after hearing our experiences, have reported similar results. On Alex's personal blog, where he shares his decks, several students from all over the world have commented on the effectiveness of Anki. One poster wrote, "Since starting Anki a few months ago my NBME practice exam scores have increased by an average of 20 points!" Similarly, the many students who've used other medicine-centric SRS platforms such as Memorang and Firecracker over the years have corroborated these sentiments.

## Spaced Repetition Software is efficient

When you're studying normally, whether it's re-reading your notes or doing review questions, you'll often find that there are many items that you already knew. As a result, although you do end up reviewing some important facts that you'd forgotten, a lot of your time is wasted rehashing things you didn't need to review. One of the strongest points of SRS is that its spacing schedule ensures that this rarely happens with your studying. If you have a fact down cold, most iterations of SRS adjust to show it to you less often. So, the only time you actually see a card is when the SRS app's scheduling algorithm predicts that you're about to forget that fact. SRS lets you cut down your studying to the minimum necessary to retain all the facts you need to know. This is a great time-savings, impossible to achieve any other way.

SRS is efficient in another way too: its mobility and flexibility allows you to study during chunks of time you couldn't have used to do desk studying. Think about the fragmented bits of time throughout your day – when you're walking to class from the parking lot, waiting in line at the grocery store, or waiting for rounds to start in the hospital. If you add up all those moments in a day, that's a lot of time that you could be studying!

SRS apps are available for most mobile devices. During the preclinical years, we could take our reviewing outside and take a walk while reviewing. During our clinical year, where large blocks of time were very rare, both of us were able to keep up with all of our daily reviews because we always had our SRS cards on our smartphones or tablets. While we could have just been standing around waiting for something interesting to happen on the wards, we were using our precious downtime to learn and review.

You have a lot of ground to cover in medical school, and you don't always have large blocks of protected time to study, especially during clinical year. So SRS's ability to let us study on the go and in little pockets of free time is extremely valuable.

## Spaced Repetition Software is flexible

SRS provides the schedule for our learning, but it's otherwise a blank slate. Any kind of knowledge that we want to retain can go in the program. Medicine is our focus, but people have used SRS to learn and remember all kinds of things, from Chinese to calculus.

SRS can use every type of medium for learning: text, audio, video, and images. Recall from *Brain Science* that people learn better from words and pictures than from words alone. SRS enables us to recruit all our senses in the learning experience since we can make cards with images, audio, and text.

The flexibility of SRS can be a double-edged sword, however, because it means that we will often have to make the cards ourselves. By itself this isn't a huge burden – it's no more work than taking notes the normal way would be. But it means that we're responsible for the quality of our cards, which in turn determines the quality of our learning and retention. Because it's important to make high quality cards to study from, we'll spend a lot of time in this section talking about how to make good cards.

## Spaced Repetition Software is digital

Think back to your college days. How many thousands of pages of printed lecture slides, outlines, and note sheets did you make? Where are they now? Sitting under your bed in a box or in a dark corner in your parents' house. So all the information you captured during those years is inaccessible.

SRS gets around this problem because it is digital and organized. SRS functions as a permanent repository of all of your notes, and you can search and find something at the tap of a button. We cannot tell you how many times we've used the search function to check a fact or to look something up. And because most SRS apps can sync into the cloud, you can be sure that your hard-earned knowledgebase is safe. That is something you can't say about paper notes.

# A large community

SRS platforms have become so popular as learning tools that there are now large and thriving user communities on the web surrounding each platform. This is important for two reasons. One is that if you ever have a question about using an SRS app, there are many people who are willing to help – we've asked questions in the forums and received prompt and informative responses. Another is that with a large user base, developers of SRS apps will continue to improve on their programs and make them even more valuable.

# SRS liberates us by making decisions for us

There's a psychological principle called the Paradox of Choice, which says that giving people more choices can sometimes make them *worse* off by promoting anxiety about making a choice. They feel regret when looking back and feel that the grass would have been greener had they chosen one of the other options. Many medical students face this with respect to their studies. They are not sure where to devote their efforts at any particular time, and wonder whether their time would be better spent shoring up anatomy or learning more pathology.

SRS helps with this by making the choices for us. Taking advantage of the spacing effect without a tool like SRS would be very challenging – we'd have to know what to review and when to review, with knowledge of the rate of decay of our own memories. But SRS takes care of that for us, serving up exactly those facts we most need to study at any given moment. All we need to do is to do the reviews that our SRS schedules for us, secure in the knowledge that the algorithm is keeping tabs on our learning.

This might sound like losing control, but actually it's very liberating. No time or effort is wasted in trying to figure out what to study. At any time, you can open up your SRS and know exactly what you need to do. And you have no excuse to procrastinate by fiddling with a study schedule. The psychic benefits are huge.

# What SRS is not

As you can tell, we think SRS is extremely valuable. But sometimes in our zeal for sharing our appreciation for SRS with other people, they infer some incorrect conclusions. So, let's dispel some misconceptions here.

## 1. You don't learn by looking at flashcards

Some people misunderstand and think we're advocating learning entirely from flashcards. On the contrary: SRS is just one piece of the equation. Looking at a bunch of flashcards is not an effective way to learn new information since there is no context, no relationship between those cards. You'll be left with an unstructured, unorganized body of facts that you'll have a hard time learning anything from.

SRS's major role is in the *retention* of information rather than the *acquisition* of new knowledge. You have to learn the material first, and then it's the job of SRS to make sure you do not forget it. Of course, this leads to the question "so how *do* I try to learn new information?" This is a topic that we will go into much greater depth on in the next section, *Learning Method.*

## 2. SRS is not the only thing you need for effective learning

SRS is the core of our learning system, but it is not the only component. As we'll discuss in the next section, there are several stages in the learning process. SRS helps with some of them, but for others, we need different tools. For example, application of knowledge is the end goal of learning. In medicine, we use practice questions, simulators, standardized patients and the like to practice applying our knowledge. SRS can enhance these activities, but it is not a replacement for them. To be a truly effective learner, you need to use multiple tools and strategies, which is what we advocate with our learning method.

# Anki – Our preferred SRS program

As we mentioned above, there are several different SRS apps, which each have their own distinct advantages and disadvantages. We explore these SRS options later in Chapter 7, but from here on out, we're going to discuss how to use our preferred SRS program, Anki.

Both of us have used Anki throughout medical school, and continue to use it today. So why did we pick Anki over other SRS programs, and why we do make it the emphasis of the forthcoming chapters? There are several reasons. First, Anki is open-source, which means that is free to use on most platforms, and that users can build custom add-ons to get more out of the program. Moreover, being open source means that the card decks belong to you and not anyone else, allowing you to do as you please with your content. Second, Anki has a lot of powerful features such as searching, tagging, various learning modes, and solid analytics to help you track your performance. Finally, Anki is available on every platform, desktop, web, and mobile, allowing you to use it everywhere.

For these reasons, we think Anki is best in class right now (early 2015). This may change; at some point in the future, a better tool may emerge. But while the tools change, the principles will be timeless. For now, let's get started using Anki.

# Chapter 5:
# Getting Started With Anki

Now that we've talked about why we use Anki, let's now walk through actually using it.

## Getting started

Download Anki from www.ankisrs.net and install it. This site has versions for Windows, Mac, Linux, as well as iPhone and Android (we'll talk about the mobile app later).

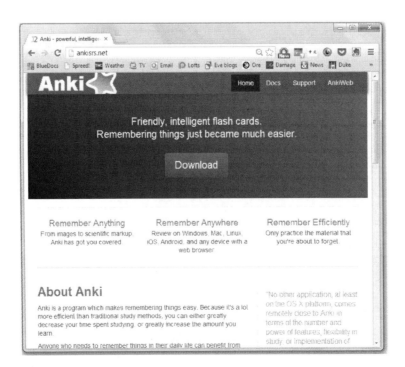

# Create your first deck

Anki's major organizer for cards is the deck. A deck is just a group of cards, usually pertaining to a certain subject. The first screen that you see when you open Anki is called the *Deck Browser* and you can see all the decks that you have.

1. Once downloaded and installed, open Anki. The first screen you'll see is the home deck browser. Right now there is just the default deck that Anki creates when you open it up for the first time. In time, there will be many more decks here.

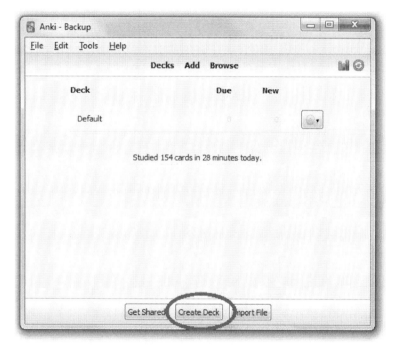

2. We're going to create a deck called "Pathology." Go ahead and click "create deck"

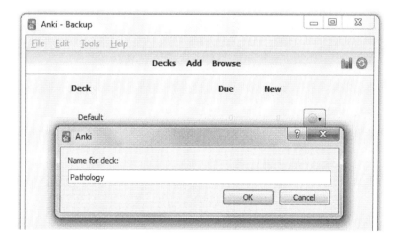

3.  Type in Pathology. There's your first deck!

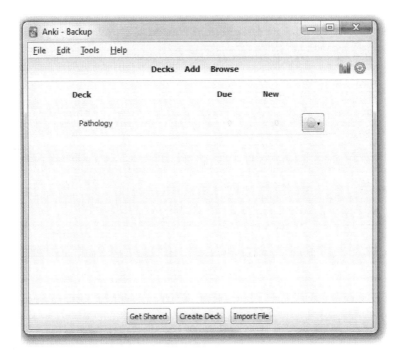

# Creating a card

Now that we have a deck, we need to fill it in with some cards. Let's create a flashcard on cardiology for our pathology deck.

1.  Open the Pathology deck by clicking on its name.

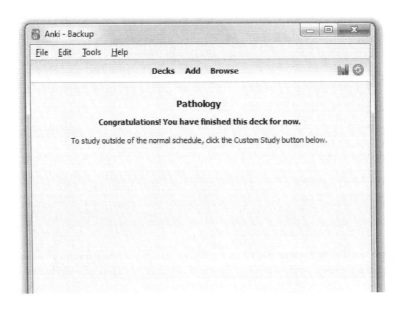

2. To create a new card, click "Add." The window that pops up lets you add new cards to your deck. You can see that there are many buttons and options on this screen, but let's not worry about that for now.

3. Let's make a card about cardiology. On the front we can write a question: What is the mechanism of aortic stenosis? On the back we have the answer: Calcification of the aortic valve. In the tag field, add the tag "cardiology" (see more below). Type all this in and hit "Add." There we have it, our first card!

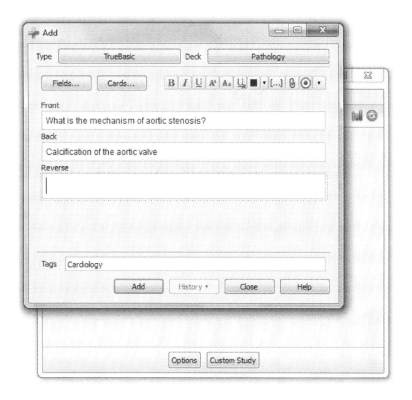

# Tagging

So let's talk about that tag we just added in Step 3 above.

In Anki, a tag is just another piece of information that helps sort and file a card. You're likely familiar with tags from blogs or note-taking program like Evernote.

Tagging becomes important when we go to do our learning and review. Right now our Pathology deck isn't exactly bursting at the seams. But as you add more cards to your decks, you'll need a way to hone in on specific subsets of all those cards. Without tagging, there would be no way to tell Anki which of those subsets you want to see.

So let's return to our cardiology card we just created. It's Sunday night, and tomorrow morning, you have a test on cardiac pathology. Your knowledge about the cardiology is a little shaky, and you want to review before the test. But at this point in the year, your Pathology deck has swollen to over 1000 cards, about all parts of the body. Right now though, you just want to look at the cards related to cardiology. So how do we do that?

Tags! You wisely added the tag "cardiology" to your cards when you created them. To see only the cards that have these tags, you can use Anki's "custom study" feature (see more below) to create a temporary deck that only shows you cards labeled "cardiology."

# Tagging best practices

The freeform nature of tagging is both a blessing and a curse. On the one hand, you can dice up your cards into as many subsets as you want. On the other hand, you don't get much direction about how to create tags that will help you study and search later on. To help you overcome this problem, we offer some guidelines for tagging.

When you create a new card, Anki looks at the "tag" box and creates a separate tag anywhere there is a space. So, for example, if in the tag tab we put **antibiotics endocarditis cardiac**, it would create three separate tags, "antibiotics," "endocarditis," and "cardiac." If we want a two-word tag, we need to use another character, like an underscore ( _ ) or hyphen (-) to separate the words. Keep in mind that Anki is case sensitive, so if you were to type "Renal_pathology" in a card, Anki would consider that a separate tag from "renal_pathology." We recommend that you always use lower case, just to avoid confusion.

Here are two major ways you might create tags:

### 1. Use the natural divisions of a subject

In many subjects in medicine, the most natural division is an organ system. So, for example, in Pathology or Physiology, tagging cards as "cardiovascular," "renal," or "gastrointestinal" is quite appropriate and aligns with the way that medical school divides up topics. Other divisions are subject specific. For example, in pharmacology, in addition to organ system, you might want tag cards based on drug class. i.e. antibiotics, antidepressants, antihypertensives.

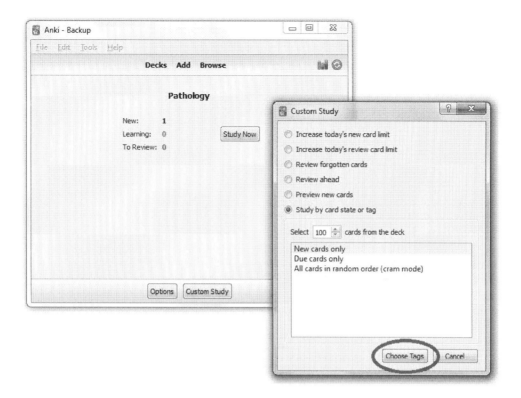

## 2. Tag cards for specific purposes

Sometimes, you may want to group cards together that are relevant to a specific goal, such as an exam. Rather than creating a new deck, it's best to use a card to group these exam-specific cards. So, for example, in our cardiology card from above, you might also add the tag "exam_5" or "cardiology_exam." The naming here isn't important, so long as it helps you categorize the cards you need to see.

# Reviewing

Now that we have the card down, let's do some studying.

1. Close the Add screen and click Study Now on the deck screen.

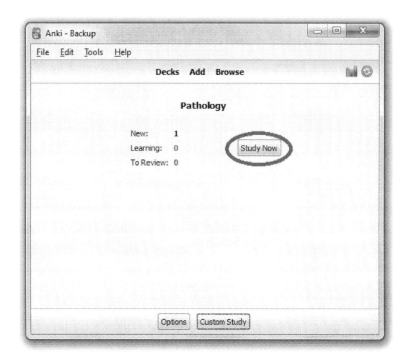

2. Now we have the question displayed: "What is the mechanism of aortic stenosis?" Do you remember the answer? Think about the answer in your head, then check your response by clicking "Show Answer."

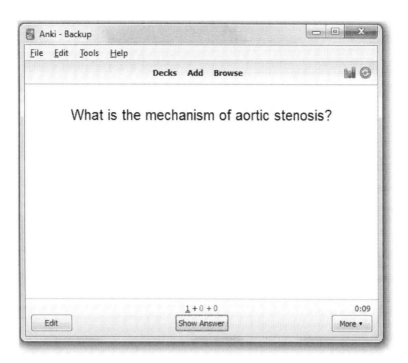

3. Check your response with the answer. If you got it wrong, click "Again." If you got it easily, click "Easy." If you were able to get it after thinking a little, click "Good." Notice that each option has a time interval associated with it; the easier a question is for you, the longer the period before you need to review it again.

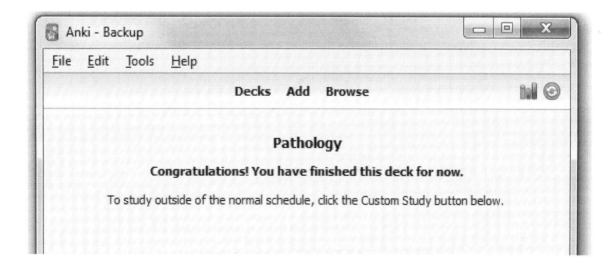

4. And with that, we're back to the deck's home screen. Our reviews are done for the day! Click Decks to return to the deck browser.

# Browse

We've only got one card so far, so it's not too hard to keep track of. But that won't be the case for long. Once you've accumulated a lot of cards, it can be difficult to hunt for a fact that want to look up. Anki's Browse function lets you search through your existing cards, both by keywords and by tags.

1. Open up the Browse screen by clicking Browse at the top of the home screen

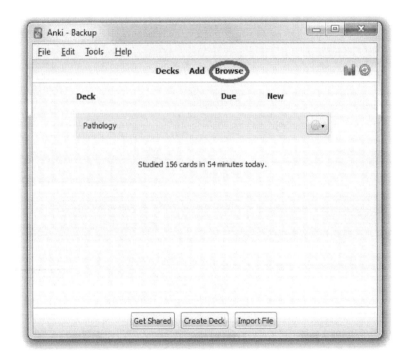

2. One way to search for cards is by keyword. Suppose we wanted to find cards that talked about cardiology. Type "aortic" into the search bar at the top of the screen, and click "Search" to see what we've got about the aorta or aortic valve. We can see our card pop up, just as expected.

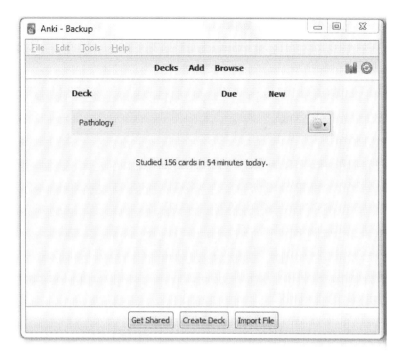

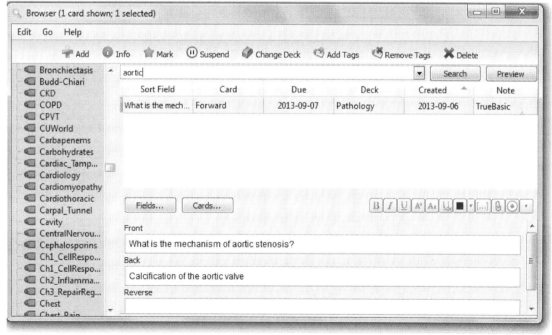

3. Another way to search for cards is by tags. We've just tagged our aortic stenosis card with "cardiology." Suppose we wanted to check over our cardiology-related cards, either for our own review or for a test coming up. Look for the tag "cardiology" on the left hand column and click on it to bring up all the cards tagged "cardiology"

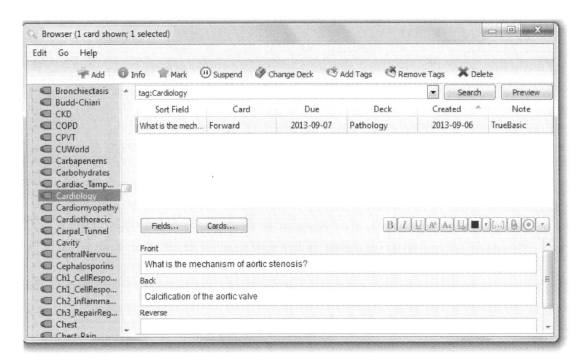

4. Within the browse screen we can modify the cards we bring up. We can change the text on the front and back, and add or remove tags. In fact, we're going to modify our aortic stenosis card right now by adding media.

# Adding media

The spacing and testing effect are powerful, but as we've discussed in the *Brain Science* section, we can improve our learning even further by incorporating audiovisual aids into our studying. Fortunately, Anki supports adding media - both picture and audio - that can augment your learning.

1. Let's go back to our aortic stenosis card. Use the Browse window to pull it up.

2. Reviewing the mechanism of aortic stenosis is all well and good, but maybe a visual aid - say, a picture of a stenotic aortic valve - would make this fact more impactful. Let's go find a picture on the Wikipedia article on aortic stenosis. Copy that picture (right-click, copy image) and paste it in the answer field of the card. Now whenever we review that fact, we will not only have information on the mechanism of aortic stenosis, we'll be reminded what it looks like.

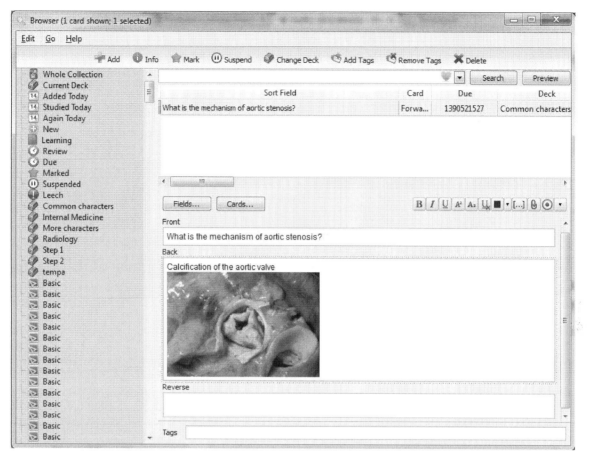

3. You can do the same thing with sound files. Aortic stenosis produces a unique murmur, which might be worth associating with this card. Search online for a sound clip of this murmur, and paste it into the card.

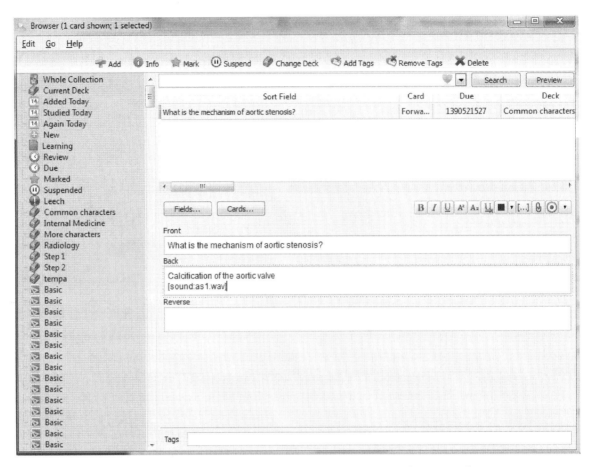

In summary, after reading this guide, you should have Anki up and running on your computer. You have learned how to create decks and review flashcards in them. You've learned a set of skills for creating cards for any topic you liked, appropriately tagged and enhanced by audiovisual aids. And finally, you'll have learned how to browse, sort, and edit your cards.

# Custom study

Sometimes your schedule places unique demands on your studying. Through the "custom study" option, Anki gives you tools to address several common scenarios.

To access custom study, open up the Pathology deck again. On the bottom right is the Custom Study button. Clicking it brings up several options. We've found two of these options to be helpful:

**Review ahead** lets you review cards due tomorrow or the day after. This option comes in handy if you have some extra time for studying today and know that you'll be too busy tomorrow to review your cards.

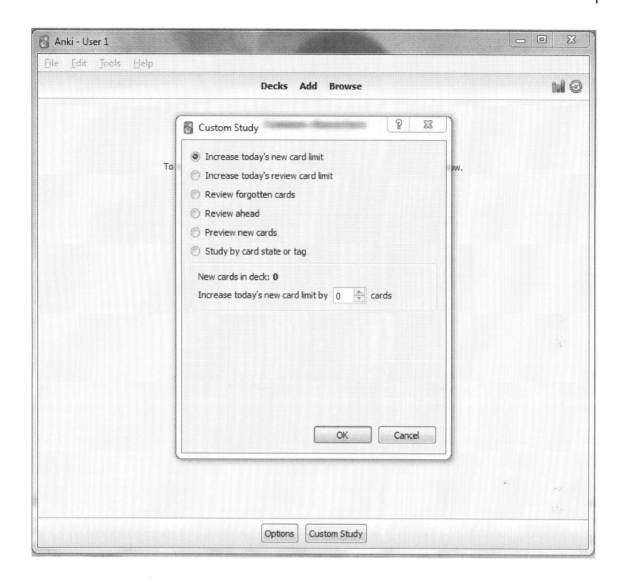

**Study by card state or tag** lets you selectively review cards with specific tags. So, for example, if you wanted to study for a cardiology exam, you might look for cards tagged "cardiology." Here is where our hard work tagging pays off! Anki calls this mode "cram mode" and that's exactly what it does – it turns our spaced repetition system into a cramming system when that's what we need.

When you choose either of these options, Anki generates a new deck containing the cards you're studying. Once you're done studying, you can delete those decks. The cards will not be deleted, but rather they'll go back to the decks they originally came from. Only with Anki could your cramming become part of your long-term learning strategy!

# I want to learn more!

This guide should be enough to get you started making and reviewing cards. But Anki has a number of other features that power users can take advantage of. We recommend getting familiar with the basic features first, using Anki for a few days and working out a workflow that works for you. Then you can dive into the online user manual and figure out how to use these advanced features to help Anki go even farther for you.

# AnkiWeb and mobile apps

Anki doesn't have to just be on your computer. There are mobile apps for both Android and iOS, and there's a cloud app as well that preserves and syncs your data across all your devices.

To get us started, let's set up an AnkiWeb account so the decks you just created will be synced to the cloud. Go to the AnkiWeb site (https://ankiweb.net/) and sign up for an account. Then open Anki on your computer and click the sync button in the upper right corner.

It will prompt you for the username and password that you just created. Once you enter it, the program will automatically upload your decks so that they can be accessed anywhere from Ankiweb or your mobile device.

Now let's get Anki working on your mobile device. If you have an iPhone or iPad, go to the Apple app store and buy the AnkiMobile app ($24.99). If you have an Android device, go to the Google Play store and buy the AnkiDroid app (free). Install the app, and again click the sync button and enter your login information. You'll have your cards ready to go.

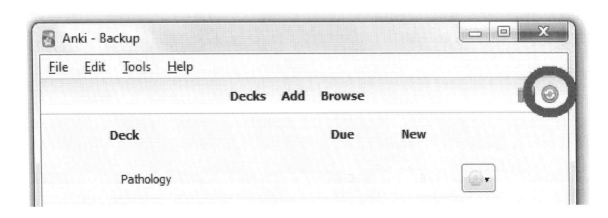

*iOS app*

*Android app*

# Chapter 6: Studying With Anki

Now that we've got the program up and running, let's talk about how we'd want to use it in the course of our study schedule.

## Daily reviews

The power of Anki lies in its ability to help us employ the spacing and testing effects. To take full advantage of that power, we should rely on Anki to schedule our daily review schedule. Every day, you will have cards that are due for review. Some of those reviews will be for things you've learned in the last few days. Others will be reviews of things you learned farther in the past. No matter when you learned them, or what your current learning demands are, if you want to get the best results, you should do all the reviews that are scheduled for you, in order to adhere as closely as possible to your personal forgetting curve.

To be sure, sometimes things come up and you can't do your reviews for the day — maybe you're traveling, or it's the day of a big exam. That's OK if it happens once in a while. But if large lapses occur, your scheduled reviews will pile up, and it will become much more difficult to work your backlog down to zero. So, you should try to minimize lapses as much as possible.

# Common pitfalls

### 1. Waiting to review new cards en masse

Some people will, incorrectly, put off reviewing new information until a later time, sometimes days later. The problem here is that those early memories from studying are transient. If your first review is not done within 24 hours of learning, you're more likely to forget what you learned and will have to go back and re-learn the material in order to answer the questions on the card. It's more efficient to do your initial reviews soon after you finished studying.

### 2. Learning too many new cards at once

There are several reasons to avoid this. One is that your brain can only take in so much new information at a time. There is no empirically defined number of new facts, but our experience and that of other Anki power users is to do no more than 100 new cards/day.

The other reason to avoid this is that you'll end up with a lot of reviews falling on the same day in the future. In the early days after you learn a card, the cards you answered correctly will have identical spacing intervals. That means that the cards you do one day will stay together, and come due together. And on that day, you'll get slammed with a bunch of reviews, which can become overwhelming. Many people who dabbled with Anki drop it at this point because they become overwhelmed with reviews. Slow and steady wins the race.

### 3. Focusing too much on card-making rather than review

Some people believe that most of the value of Anki is in the making of the flashcards. This is not true. Yes, there is some value in card-making since it forces you to pay attention and read with a judicious eye. But the magic of Anki, and spaced repetition in general, is in the retrieval – that is, in the actual reviewing of the cards. Remember that the act of retrieval itself alters and augments memories, making them stronger and more connected to other bits of information. So if you can get high-quality premade cards, or collaborate with classmates to create decks, you're saving time and still capturing the majority of the value from Anki. Don't turn that down.

# How to make good cards

Anki can be helpful even if you just start using it without any further instruction. But there are common pitfalls, especially when it comes to making Anki cards. Done well, your flashcards can be invaluable aids to memory; done poorly, they can be little better than cumbersome electronic note sheets. Here are some key principles to ensure your cards are pulling their weight.

## One fact per card

Many people think of a flashcard as a 3 x 5 index card with lots of information scribbled on it. For example, you might have seen people make paper flashcards with "S. Aureus" on the front, and then on the back, a dozen facts about *S. Aureus*. When you make them this way, flashcards are nothing more than mobile textbook clippings. Their portability might be a plus, but otherwise, there is nothing special about them. Flashcards for spaced repetition share the same name as these paper versions, but serve a completely different purpose.

Let's say you made the following card:

Q: How does *S. aureus* differ from other staphylococci?
A: Coagulase positive. Metabolizes maltose. Beta-hemolytic. Has protein A.

The card has one prompt, and a lot of related facts. But here's the problem. What if you answered the card with "has protein A and metabolizes maltose." You'd be partially right, but partially wrong as well. How do you score such an answer? The two things you got right you don't need to review; the ones you got wrong need more study. But because those bits of info are on the same card, there is no way for you to accurately rate the card. Either you count that as correct, in which case you wouldn't get to review the two facts you missed, or you count it as incorrect, in which case you'd waste time reviewing the two facts you already knew.

Remember that our goal is to use these cards to take advantage of the spacing effect and the testing effect. In order for to make use of the spacing effect, we need to be able to accurately evaluate our performance for each fact we learn. The only way to do that consistently and accurately is to only put one fact – one question/answer pair – per card.

The right way to learn about *S. aureus* would be to make four different cards, one for each factoid:

Q: How does *S. aureus* differ from other staphylococci with respect to coagulase?
A: *S. Aureus* is coagulase positive; rest are coagulase negative.

Q: How does *S. aureus* differ from other staphylococci with respect to maltose digestion?
A: *S. Aureus* digests maltose; rest do not

You get the idea. Yes, making these flashcards will take a little more work, but now you can learn each of these facts, rather than being hobbled by unwieldy cards that won't let you learn all four facts. In the long run your effort will be well worth it. So whenever and wherever possible, we should aim to break information down into the smallest possible question/answer pair.

Here's another example.

**Wrong:**
Q: Ejection fraction
A: Index of ventricular contractility. Normally >55%, decreased in heart failure.

**Right:**
Q: What does ejection fraction measure?
A: Ventricular contractility

Q: What is the normal value for ejection fraction?
A: >55%

Q: What happens to ejection fraction in heart failure?
A: Decreased

# Be specific

Quick, answer this question:

Q: Pancreatitis

Huh? The problem with this card is clear: it's not specific. The question doesn't give you any idea what information you're asking for. Are you looking for the causes of pancreatitis, the clinical presentation, or the treatment? Let's look at the rest of the card:

Q: Pancreatitis
A: Epigastric abdominal pain radiating to back, anorexia, nausea

Okay, so we're looking for three symptoms of pancreatitis. Now, if you *had* to learn this flashcard, you could theoretically memorize the answer to give when you see this pancreatitis question. So, whenever you see "pancreatitis" you'd have to remember that you're being asked to recall three symptoms of pancreatitis, even though the question stem doesn't tell you that. But here's the problem: this means that you have to memorize two facts instead of one! You have to memorize the symptoms of pancreatitis, as well as remembering what exactly it means when you see a question with the stem of "Pancreatitis."

You can halve your burden of memorization by simply ensuring that each of your cards has a question that clearly states the fact that you're meant to recall. Your question should say exactly what the answer is supposed to cover. And if the answer is in the form of a list, say exactly how many items are on that list. That way, you can focus your efforts on learning the medicine you're trying to learn. Here's how you might rewrite the pancreatitis card:

> Your question should say exactly what the answer is supposed to cover.

Q: Pancreatitis: 3 cardinal symptoms
A: Epigastric abdominal pain radiating to back, anorexia, nausea

# Dealing with lists

Medicine is full of lists: differential diagnoses, clinical presentations, and lab result patterns. As a result, we do often have to make an exception to "One fact per card." When you have to use lists, there are two techniques that can help make them more manageable.

First, whenever possible, you should combine related items to reduce the burden of memorization. The difficulty of remembering any list increases exponentially with the number of items. Here's an example:

Q: Digoxin side effects (4)
A: Nausea, diarrhea, blurry yellow vision, vomiting

After:

Q: Digoxin side effects (3)
A: Nausea/vomiting, diarrhea, blurry yellow vision

Secondly, use mnemonics. They may sound silly, but mnemonics can help organize a long list of items into a single memory unit. This will both help you remember each particular item on the list, as well as ensuring that you remember the list as a whole. For example, a mnemonic for the pituitary hormones if "FLAT PiG", which stands for **F**ollicle-Stimulating Hormone, **L**uteinizing Hormone, **A**drenocorticotropic Hormone, **T**hyroid-Stimulating Hormone, **P**rolactin, **i**gnore and **G**rowth Hormone. Using mnemonics combined with Anki can be very powerful.

# Use images

Humans are visual – a quarter of our brain is dedicated to visual processing, compared to the paltry portion assigned to verbal and abstract reasoning. And a lot of medicine is visual – anatomic relationships, biochemical pathways, histologic features. Using images liberally can help to cement key facts in your mind, whether it's anatomic relationships or physical exam findings.

# Image occlusion

One technique to take this one step further is to make the image the question itself. We do this by image occlusion. Simply put, take an image of something you want to memorize and use Paint to black out a key structure or metabolite. This goes in the question field of the card; the answer is the original image. Again, we don't want to ask too many questions on a single card, so only block out one or two items that you want to quiz yourself on. (You can make multiple versions of the same card, blocking out different items.) We'll go into much greater detail when in the Anatomy chapter of the *Implementation* section, but for now here is an example of how an image occlusion card might look:

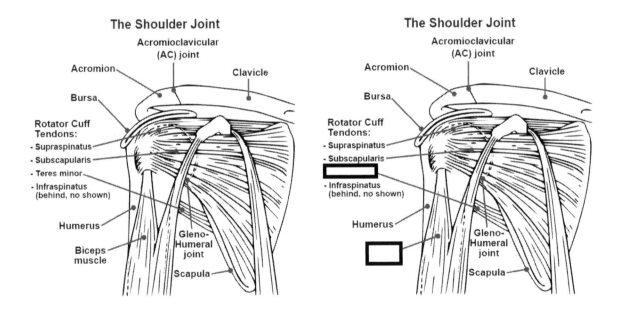

# Keep it short

You want to spend as much of your study time as possible testing yourself and practicing retrieval of knowledge. Long-winded questions and answers detract from that by making you read long passages before you get to test yourself. Cut down on this by making both questions and answers as concise as possible. "Everything should be as simple as possible, but not simpler."

# Do not memorize if you do not understand

We've mentioned it before, but this point bears repeating. Anki is a tool for maintaining and deepening memory. It is *not* a tool for learning. So as you study, first learn the subject in question and wrap your head around its entirety. Then, and only then, break it down into single, granular questions and plug them into Anki.

# What's card-worthy?

There's a short answer and a long answer to this question. The short answer is: if your studying is geared towards going well on the boards, you can confidently rely on First Aid as a guide on what's worth making a card out of. Follow along with First Aid as you're learning anything – not as a primary learning tool, but as a reference for what facts are boards-worthy. If the factoid in question is in First Aid, or helps you learn something in First Aid (say, by explaining the mechanism by which a disease has its effects), then put it in Anki. If not, it's not worth making a card out of.

The longer answer is that you'll want to make a card for whatever is worth putting in long-term memory. Anki is a great tool for retaining information in your long-term memory. But not everything has to go in there. There are some things you don't need in Anki because you'll see them frequently enough on your own to memorize them without its help. For example, you probably know your own email address because you've had to type it in repeatedly and thereby cement it in your memory. The same is true of some medical facts too; you likely know that pneumonia is an infection of the lung, and if not, that will be hammered into you enough without needing to resort to Anki.

On the opposite extreme, there are things that are rare enough that you'll never really need to have it in your memory; it's enough to know that it's something you can look up. I don't know the capital of Tajikistan, but I know I can always find it on Wikipedia. In the medical realm you may not know the tumor staging algorithm for thyroid cancer, but unless you're an oncologist you won't need to have it memorized; you can look it up if it ever comes up while still providing equally good care.

The important things to put in Anki, then, are the things that are in between – they don't come to your attention frequently enough to trigger memory, but *do* come up frequently enough that you need to have them in mind when the situation arises. As a rule of thumb, you'll spend about five minutes over the course of your lifetime reviewing each card. So, if you'll likely spend more than five minutes in your lifetime looking up a fact, it's worth making a card.

# Make your own cards or buy pre-made?

As more medical students are realizing the benefits of an SRS, the following question inevitably arises: "Should I make my own cards or use someone else's?"

This is an important question, and there are pros and cons to either option. Making your own cards is not an exceptionally hard thing to do. It's comparable to the burden of taking conventional notes. When you make your own cards, you can control exactly what goes in, and you know that you are getting high quality cards tailored to your needs. Nevertheless, it is work that takes time, and while you do get a little learning from the process of writing things down, it doesn't compare to the efficiency of actually using the flashcards.

The ideal situation would be that a source comes bundled with high-quality SRS notes/cards that correspond to the content in the source. You'd have a textbook, say *BRS Physiology*, that comes with a well-made Anki deck that corresponds to the information found in the text, just like textbooks now come with back-of-the-chapter practice questions. You could just read the textbook with the confidence that the necessary flashcards would be waiting for you at the end.

Sadly, this kind of bundled resource does not yet exist. Hopefully one day it will, and we are keeping a close eye on the online services that are beginning to provide pre-made flashcards (we'll address these in the next chapter.) But in the meantime, we have some options that can reduce or eliminate the burden of making your own SRS cards.

- Collaborate with your classmates to distribute the burden of making SRS cards/notes.
- Use SRS decks from upperclassmen that were made for specific purposes. This is akin to how upperclassmen will pass down class notes and other resources that pertained to specific exams and the like.
- Use a commercial source such as Firecracker, Memorang or Osmosis. See the next chapter for a more detailed discussion about these sources.

# Chapter 7:
## Other Spaced Repetition Software

Anki is our program of choice for learning using spaced repetition, and this is why we've gone into such detail about how to set it up and get the most use out of it. However, spaced repetition is a general principle and can be employed in a number of ways. In recent years, several companies have started producing their own spaced repetition offerings. Some are general and content-agnostic, much like Anki. Others, such as Firecracker and Osmosis, are specific to medicine and come with their own pre-loaded content.

Although Anki is the program that we've come to know and trust, we are keeping a close eye as the field of spaced repetition tools for medicine continues to expand. We've tried out several of the new services out there, and have even sat down to talk with some several of the founders of the companies. Here are some examples of the alternatives available today. They all have their pros and cons, but any of these tools can be used with our learning system. Keep in mind that these assessments are a snapshot in time. Many of these services are young startups and their offerings may have changed since the writing of this book. Thus, we encourage you to seriously consider these other SRS platforms to see whether they best fit your specific needs and preferences.

# Content-agnostic SRS programs

## Brainscape

This is a program very similar to Anki. As with Anki, it uses a spaced repetition algorithm to decide what flashcards you study. There is a desktop program and a mobile app, and you can create flashcards on your own. Alternatively, the site offers decks for sale, from foreign language vocabulary to coding shortcuts for several programming languages. Currently, they don't offer any medical flashcards for sale, so there is no reason to prefer it over Anki for now. The one advantage you may find is that Brainscape's iOS version is free, whereas Anki charges $25 (as the only revenue source for the project.) However, you have to weigh the fact that Anki is open source and a much longer-lived project; with Brainscape (and many of these newer companies) you'll be taking the risk that the app may not be supported if the company goes under or radically changes its strategy. Overall, we don't recommend using Brainscape for now, but it may be worth checking in periodically to see if they've started offering high quality, medically relevant flashcards.

## Cerego

Now for something different. This is a flashcard program that uses spaced repetition, but unlike Anki, which asks you how well you remember something and takes your response on trust, Cerego actually creates a mini quiz with each card. It asks you to choose the correct answer among several answers randomly drawn from your flashcards. This is a neat trick, and works well with Cerego's collection of premade cards. Indeed, the company has partnered with Elsevier and other publishers to create many decks of variable quality.

However, this quizzing approach makes it a lot harder to create your own decks. After all, the multiple-choice quiz format makes sense only if all the questions in a deck have similar formats. If you had drug names, physiology responses, and anatomic structures all mixed together in a deck, the format would no longer makes sense; the answer would be too obvious. Cerego might be a useful supplement if you're looking for premade decks and find some high quality ones, but it's not as flexible as Anki to be a backbone of your learning system.

## Supermemo

This is the granddaddy of modern spaced repetition software. First created in 1985, it has similar features to Anki and is available in desktop and mobile versions. However, unlike Anki, development on this project hasn't been very active. It's also not free – the latest version costs $60. So we don't particularly recommend it when compared to Anki, but it does at least use the same spaced repetition algorithm.

## Mnemosyne

This is another fully general flash card program using a spaced repetition algorithm. However, unlike the other alternatives listed, it doesn't currently have a mobile version for iOS. In a world where smartphones and tablets are so prevalent, this is a significant weakness, and we therefore don't recommend using this program.

# Medicine-specific programs

## Firecracker

Previously known as Gunner Training, this website pairs a spaced repetition algorithm with thousands of questions based based on high-yield content for USMLE Step 1 and Step 2CK. You can review questions on the website, or on its mobile apps. The website is subscription-based, with a current cost of $39 a month or $399 a year.

The greatest strength of this website is that the cards are already made for you. They're reasonably high-quality, and taken largely from from reputable sources. You can also add your own cards and make notes on existing cards. There are significant limitations here, however. The yearly cost is pretty steep, and you can't take the paid content with you after your subscription lapses. This means that if you are planning to use your cards for lifetime learning, Firecracker may not be the best choice. However, Firecracker would be a solid choice for people who are planning to study just for Step 1, and aren't planning to continue using their cards afterwards. If you're interested in spaced repetition but really don't want to make your own content, Firecracker is a good alternative.

## Memorang

This is a relatively new SRS platform that's created a great deal of content in a short amount of time. Like the other services, Memorang is built on a backbone of spaced repetition, and has both desktop and mobile versions. The core service is free and lets you make your own cards; the site makes money by subscription access to premade cards for Step 1 and Step 2 CK, as well as some other exams. (Current prices are $9 per month, $59 per year for each test.) An important advantage over Anki is the ease of collaborating with your classmates on building decks. While Anki allows collaboration as well, Memorang's web-based interface makes collaborative deck building much simpler. There are a few additional features worth noting here. In addition to flashcard format, the site also allows students to do multiple-choice questions and matching questions, similar to Cerego. Importantly, no matter what review method you use, you get the same spaced repetition algorithm keeping track of your learning, so none of your efforts are wasted.

In contrast to Anki and many of the other SRS apps, which use an expanding interval schedule, Memorang currently uses what they call a "session-based" spaced repetition. According to their blog, this mode of spaced repetition aims to help learners master information in a short period of time, as opposed to making a schedule for long-term retention using ever-expanding intervals. Because this format is new, we cannot say how it compares to the more traditional expanding interval schedule of Anki and other SRS apps, although we suspect it will be better for students with more immediate goals rather than those who want to retain for the long term. Memorang has announced that it will release a schedule-based system that prompts reviews at pre-determined times, but that option is not available now, unfortunately.

Nevertheless, this is definitely an up and coming service with a lot of potential. As with Firecracker, it's a good choice for students who either don't want to make, or don't have the time to make their own cards, and are not interested in pursuing retention of that knowledge after test day.

# Osmosis

This service is a little different than the previous two. It functions as a hybrid between a question bank and traditional class notes, all with a spaced repetition engine in the background. It provides pre-made flashcards and in its paid version, lets you submit your lecture slides and class notes and allow the site to extract the text to find flashcards and other learning aids relevant to the topic. They also built in social features so that you can collaborate with your classmates and share tips based on the latest lectures. As with the other subscription services, you gain from not having to create your own flashcards, but lose from no longer having access once your subscription lapses. However, the collaborative features for Osmosis are a definite selling point.

# Chapter 8:
## Your Other Peripheral Brain – Note-Taking Systems

Anki works great for facts you want to memorize for the long term. But what about for everything else? In many cases, you'll run into facts that you don't want to spend the long-term effort to memorize, but still want to record so that you can still refer to it as needed. This is where having a note-taking system can come in handy.

There are a few cases where taking notes can make sense. The simplest case is information that you want to capture now so that you can put it into Anki later. On rounds, for instance, a resident might give you a high-yield piece of information. You aren't in front of your computer to make a flash card right then and there, but if you scribble down a note and look at it when you get home, you'll be able to save it into Anki.

Sometimes, you'll want to take notes for things you want to cram, but don't need to commit to long-term memory. For example, maybe before Step 1 you're looking to memorize some obscure chromosomal translocations that have shown up on exam questions. You're not planning to memorize them, you just want to cram them before the test and forget them afterwards. In that case, it's worth jotting down the information on paper, practice retrieving the information a few times, and leave it at that.

Finally, there may be information that you don't need to memorize, but still want to refer to later – it's not something you want to lose access to forever. For example, a lecturer might mention an interesting study that you'd like to learn more about later. You don't need to memorize the study, but you do want to save it for future reference.

For the first two cases, paper and pencil is usually a pretty good way to record information. In the third scenario, however, paper and pencil starts to show some limitations.

Think about how many notes you've taken back in college classes. Most of them are probably sitting in a basement somewhere. And even if you had them at hand, there's no way for you to easily search through them. If you wanted to find your organic chemistry notes on decarboxylation when you're learning biochem, it would be a pretty laborious process.

That's why some students have turned to electronic note systems to manage this long-term repository of information. Some students have used Evernote, a program that syncs across your phone and computer, and can input pictures as well as links and text. Google Docs is also popular, especially for short-term note-taking. There are many other options, including Drafts and nvALT for Macs, but the key is to pick a system you like and stick to it.

Finally, don't get obsessive about capturing every possible fact. Upon deliberation, you may decide that you don't need to have certain fact in permanent storage after all. Often it's more important just to know where we can look up the necessary knowledge. Once you know that, you're done – move on to the next topic you need to learn.

# Section III
## Learning Method

# Chapter 9:
## Learning Method – An Overview

So far, we've talked about the science of learning and we've introduced you to our core tool for knowledge retention, spaced repetition software (SRS). In this section of the book, we'll move from theory to practice, explaining how to put these principles and tools into action. In particular, we'll give you a flexible and effective **Learning Method** that is grounded in both evidence and experience.

We're presenting an idealized workflow that you can use to study any subject in medicine and beyond. We don't view these prescriptions as absolute. You should use this learning method as a base from which to experiment. You may need to omit or modify some elements to suit your school's time constraints, and you might find special tactics useful for certain topics. In the next section of the book, *Implementation*, we'll suggest specific ways to tailor this workflow to each subject and setting in medical school.

So let's dive in. To help guide the discussion of our Learning Method, take a look at the following diagram.

Our Learning Method consists of three major steps, represented by the blue rectangles: Acquire, Review, and Apply. Dashed lines represent the flow of information between these steps. Solid arrows represent the workflow: you first acquire information, then review it, then apply it. At the center we have our peripheral brain, which is divided into two parts: Spaced Repetition Software (SRS) and Personal Notes.

Now, let's go through the Learning Method step by step.

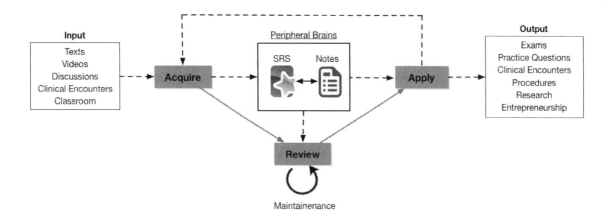

# Acquire – Taking in new information

**Acquire** is the first step in the Learning Method. This is the critical step where new information enters our minds from the outside world. We've listed just a few of the main sources you can acquire from – texts, videos, clinical encounters – but there are certainly others.

Our main goal during the Acquire step is to optimize our intake of new information and decide whether we want to commit it to memory. In the *Brain Science* section, we explored the factors that are important for the encoding and storage of new information, things like organization, priming, meaning-making, visual imagery. Here, we'll be putting these strategies to work to maximize new learning.

# Review – Making learning last

You know by now that is not enough to just be exposed to information a single time, at least not if you want to remember something for the long haul.

Accordingly, the **Review** step, with SRS at its core, is the lynchpin of our learning method. It is the step that most people do not do, resulting in temporary gains and wasted effort. By reviewing the right way, you will avoid this fate and build durable knowledge.

Let's dig in a little further. In the diagram above, you'll notice a couple of different arrows linking to review. The red arrow from Acquire to Review reflects the sequential nature of these two steps; you first need to acquire in order to have something to review. The dashed arrow leading from your peripheral brain to review indicates the flow of information from your SRS (the cues that are on your cards) into your mind. The solid arrow looping around review symbolizes maintenance reviewing. Recall from our discussion of

Spaced Repetition Software that the effectiveness of these tools comes from continuous and regular use. Causal, sporadic use brings some benefit, but much less than that which comes with consistent and daily practice.

# Apply – From theory to practice

Knowledge and learning are good things in themselves, but we're not just learning for learning's sake. We want to do something. We want to apply our knowledge toward achieving our goals. In the **Apply** step, we bring to bear the things we've learned to do something useful.

As medical learners in the classroom, applying typically means taking tests, doing practice problems and simulations, working in groups with classmates, and sometimes a creative project of some sort. As we move from the classroom to the wards, applying then takes on new meaning. It encompasses clinical tasks such as performing a physical exam, taking a patient history, giving an oral presentation on rounds, and engaging in clinical problem solving. As full-fledged physicians, applying our knowledge to patient care becomes our highest aim. Along the way, we may also utilize our knowledge for other endeavors such as research, teaching or entrepreneurship.

In the diagram above, we can see that the information we draw from comes from two sources: our long-term memory, which we have been priming with the previous steps, and our external references. On the wards, for instance, our decision-making comes from integrating our medical knowledge with external references such as UpToDate. We can set ourselves up for success by acquiring and aeviewing in a systematic way.

At the same time, applying can also be a source of information. When we apply knowledge in novel settings, we almost always pick up new information too. On the wards, both students and physicians are constantly exposed to new information with every patient encounter. In the act of applying what you know, you often also take in new information, modifying and adding to your fund of knowledge

# Reflecting – Putting the pieces together and monitoring our progress

There is one final component to the Learning Method: **Reflect**. Reflect is not a discrete step like the others because it is everywhere. Reflecting should happen while acquiring, reviewing and applying, so it doesn't fit into any particular spot in the sequence.

Recall from the *Brain Science* section that thinking hard about what you've learned is an important factor for building long-term knowledge. We discussed how connected knowledge, that which has meaning and organization, is easier to store and retrieve than disordered knowledge. We also explored how critically appraising your knowledge and your performance provides important **feedback** that you can use to improve your future learning. Reflect accomplishes all these goals; we order our thinking, we make connections, and we get useful feedback.

At each particular step, the exact mechanics of reflecting will differ slightly, but overall, the point is to think deeply and critically. During the uptake of new knowledge (Acquire), reflecting consists of connecting what you're learning to what you already know and checking for gaps in understanding. Specific, evidence-backed tactics like Self-Explanation, which we'll discuss further in this section, can be particularly helpful during this time.

During Review, you should also reflect. You should think about how the facts on your flashcards fit together. When you get questions wrong, you shouldn't just glance at the answer and move on. You should stop and think about how the correct answer differs from the one you gave, and you should consciously update your knowledge in this way.

When you're Applying, reflection is also critical, because you can use the feedback to identify gaps in your knowledge and devise a plan for improving your future performance. This kind of feedback-reflection cycle is an essential component of Deliberate Practice, which is a powerful tool toward developing expertise.[1,2]

You can see how important reflection is in each of these steps. As we go through the three core steps of the learning method in the following sections, we'll also discuss specific ways to practice reflecting.

# Preliminaries

We know you're probably itching to try out the Learning Method. But we need to do some preparation first to set ourselves up for highly effective learning. All of the steps of the Learning Method – Acquire, Review, and Apply – require you to prepare by first doing the following steps:

- Define your goals
- Make a plan
- Gather the right resources
- Focus
- Think and Organize

In this chapter, we're going to walk you through each of these steps. We'll explain how they work and why each one is important to help you make the best use of your studying efforts.

# Define your goals

People come into medical school with various academic goals. Most all of us want to learn to be a great doctor someday. In the meantime, you want to do well on the board exams and pass the test next Monday. A study plan for one goal won't necessarily help you with the other – even if you want to do orthopedics, all the musculoskeletal anatomy studying in the world won't help you pass your test on microbiology. So before we get into study strategies, let's figure out what our goals are.

For many of us, the goal is to get into a competitive residency program. You may be coming to med school knowing what you want to do, or maybe you're waiting to see what the different clinical rotations are like before making a decision. Either way, it's pretty valuable to be a strong applicant, so that you can freely choose what specialty to practice and what residency program to attend.

Fortunately, there's pretty solid data about what it takes to become a strong applicant. Green *et al.* surveyed residency directors in all specialties. They found that the most important criteria for residency selection were, in decreasing order:[3]

1. Grades in clinical clerkships
2. USMLE Step 1 score
3. Grades in senior electives in specialty
4. Number of honors grades in clerkships
5. USMLE Step 2 score

For our discussion, we've condensed down three broad goals that most every medical student will have.

1. Learning for school: focus on school's requirements
2. Learning for boards: focus on USMLE board examinations
3. Learning for life: focus on core, durable medical knowledge and skills for residency and beyond

In an ideal world, our learning efforts would satisfy all our goals at once. We'd hit all three birds with one stone, every time. In the real world, however, there's only partial overlap.

Therefore, there's tension between our different goals, and we must each decide how we prioritize our efforts. As a general rule, aim to satisfy multiple goals simultaneously, the more the better. When that's not possible, you must decide which goals are more important than others and allocate your time and energy proportionally.

For this book, we have our own priorities: while we recognize the importance of paying our dues to school and boards, we give precedence to learning for life. So, our learning efforts might look like this:

- Learning for all three goals at the same time: 60%
- Learning just for life: 20%
- Learning just for school: 10%
- Learning just for boards: 10%

Of course, this ranking and allocation will change over time, as our circumstances dictate. You should re-evaluate often and be mindful about how you allocate your time because this will in turn determine how, what and how much you study.

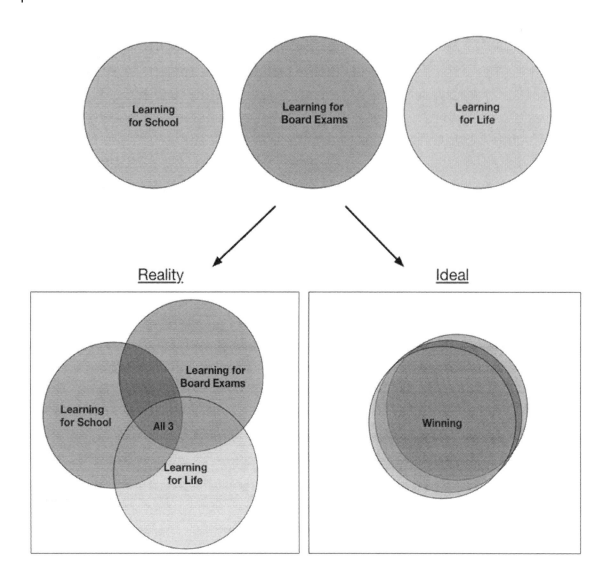

After you finish reading this section, write out your own rank list and make some estimates about how you'll want to allocate your time.

## Learning for school

Every medical school has a unique curriculum and accompanying requirements. Depending on the school, the hoops that students have to jump through may be very onerous or relatively loose. Learning for school is learning for the purpose of meeting and surpassing the requirements of your medical school. At minimum, that means passing class exams and other assessments, and at most it means performing at a very high level on everything. When learning for school, you'll be studying the topics emphasized in your school's curriculum, with the primary aim of doing well on school tests.

If you're a student at a medical school, first and foremost, you need to be concerned with getting through medical school. If you're flunking classes or not completing requirements, no matter how smart or devoted to medicine you are, you cannot become a physician.

This is all common sense, we know. But sometimes in their zeal to 'do their own thing' and learn efficiently, some students disregard their school's requirements. We've seen it happen and we don't want that for you. So, remember – you got to at least pass med school!

Thankfully, most medical schools have curricula and support systems that make failing quite difficult. Diligence, discipline, and knowing when and how to ask for help can get you through – and if you're reading this book, you almost certainly have these qualities.

That brings us to the question of how much you should care about learning for school *beyond* merely passing. Every medical school has a unique curriculum. They all contain a similar core body of knowledge, but there is significant variability between schools, both in terms of content and quality. A common complaint from medical students is that their classes focus too much on PhD-level esoterica and not enough on clinically useful information. In a similar vein, many students feel that their schools don't focus enough on preparing them for career-determining board exams.

There is no doubt that many schools do have an inordinate focus on the arcane, and that at times, students unnecessarily have to focus on regurgitating factoids about a professor's pet research interest. But med school curricula do contain a lot of useful knowledge that you will want to know and retain for a lifetime. Our advice is to take what you can from the best parts of med school and cram and forget the minutiae. Focus on the parts that align best with your longer-term goals. So many students reflexively strive for superior performance on whatever task is put before them, without thinking about if doing so will actually help them – and what they're giving up in the pursuit.

### Preclinical Grades

How much effort you devote to your preclinical grades depends on your school's grading scheme, your long-term career aspirations, and your personality. Some schools are pass/fail in the preclinical years, while others keep a traditional grading system.

If your school is pass/fail, we recommend that you take advantage of that gift and don't worry too much about your grades other than passing. Note, we're not saying be a slacker. You came to medical school to learn. But pass/fail recognizes that you're an adult and that you're capable of determining what is worth your time to learn. Glean the useful things from your school's curriculum, but use the extra time afforded to you by pass/fail to explore areas of medicine that you find meaningful and interesting. You should be the driver of your own learning.

If you don't have the luxury of pass/fail, your situation is different. You may need to be more concerned with grades, if for no other reason than that it is harder to pass (if graded on a curve relative to your classmates). But you should still give serious thought as to whether trying to ace class exams is worth the effort. Consider your longer-term goals and think about whether high performance on your school's exams will actually help you achieve them.

We can tell you from experience that there are diminishing returns when you are studying just for school. To perform at the highest levels, you need to put in an inordinate amount of effort and you get very little back for it, other than bragging rights. And, while fun, bragging rights don't translate well beyond medical school.

The thought of not aiming for 100% is foreign to most medical students, since it took an unwavering pursuit of high grades to get into med school in the first place. Even if your school has grades in the preclinical year, you should consider aiming for less than 100% for a few reasons. First, you free up valuable time to pursue your other medical and life interests, such as learning for boards and learning for life. Second, the material you'll need to learn to get top grades is usually minimally useful and will likely be forgotten. (Quick: which protein domain enables binding to phosphotyrosine residues on receptor tyrosine kinases?). Finally, from a practical standpoint, preclinical grades are of low importance to residency directors. Remember from the Green study cited above that while clinical clerkship grades do matter, preclinical don't even show up on the top five.

On the other hand, aiming for curve-breaking scores on class exams might be a worthwhile goal if:

1. **You want to get into an ultra-competitive residency:** Among the top applicants to competitive residencies, every distinction helps. The residency selection criteria survey we mentioned above does refer to preclinical grades, but it's way down the pecking order at number 12.

2. **You want to get into Alpha Omega Alpha (AOA) honor society:** This is related to the last point. For competitive residencies, AOA can be an important distinction. For example, in *Charting Outcomes in the Match* (2011), 51% of all matched applicants into dermatology were AOA, as were 46% of matched plastic surgery residents. So if you know you want to apply to a competitive residency, or if you're not sure and want to keep those doors open, your preclinical grades – and thus, you AOA prospects – will matter.

3. **You get satisfaction from being at the top:** All of us got to medical school by taking pride in our academic prowess and desiring to be 'the best' at some point in our careers. And for some medical students, pursuit of being in the nth percentile in their class or breaking the curve is a prime goal. Many won't admit it openly, but we won't knock this. Everyone is driven by something different. So if aiming for the top brings you satisfaction, be open about that with yourself, embrace it and use it to power your studying, but stay humble and graceful in that pursuit.

Summing it all up, our general recommendation is that you definitely focus on passing your school's requirements. If your school's pass/fail, that's the end of the matter, and you should be trying to learn efficiently for boards or for life instead of squeezing out an extra point on the exam. And even if your school is graded, consider whether it's really worthwhile (or possible) to try for honors in every subject, given the relative unimportance of preclinical grades and the tradeoffs you'll have to make in terms of long-term learning. If you want to aim for top grades on school stuff make sure you can tell yourself why you want to do this, and how it aligns with your other professional and personal goals.

### Clerkship grades

Let's briefly touch on clinical clerkship grades. As the Green *et al.* paper makes clear, clinical clerkship grades do matter. Indeed, they are the top criterion that residency directors cited. Given this importance, we think all medical students should strive for their personal best when on the wards. The best source of information as to how to get top marks on clerkships is from the upperclassmen at your school. Therefore, later in the book, we won't have a lot to say about what to do to excel on the wards, grade-wise. But in terms of deciding your goals and prioritizing them, the same process as we've applied to the preclinical years works:

1. Be honest with yourself about your aspirations and your abilities.
2. Clearly articulate and prioritize your learning and academic goals.
3. Pick your battles wisely. Trying to honor every clerkship is a high stress endeavor for most students. Invest the effort where it counts (i.e. in the clerkship that you're interested in matching in).
4. Review and adapt your goals to the changing circumstances.

## Learning for Board Examinations

To become a physician in the United States, any aspiring doctor must pass each of the three (actually four) steps of the USMLEs – Step1, Step2CS/CK and Step 3. You may already know what these exams are about, but let's clarify what each address.

### Step 1

*What's tested*: Basic science learned during the pre-clinical years of medical school. According to the official website, the exam "assesses whether you understand and can apply important concepts of the sciences basic to the practice of medicine, with special emphasis on principles and mechanisms underlying health, disease and modes of therapy."

*When to take it*: Usually after the end of pre-clinical year, just before the beginning of clinical year (right after 2nd year for most medical students).

### Step 2 CK

*What's tested*: Clinical knowledge acquired during clinical clerkships. The exam "assesses whether you can apply medical knowledge, skills, and understanding of clinical science essential for the provision of patient care under supervision and includes emphasis on health promotion and disease prevention."

*When to take it*: After the clinical year (3rd year for most students) and before entering residency. Most students take this exam near the end of the clinical year or early during the 4th year.

### Step 2 CS

*What's tested*: Clinical skills, using standardized patients and clinical scenarios. The exam "assesses the ability of examinees to apply medical knowledge, skills, and understanding of clinical science essential for the provision of patient care under supervision, and includes emphasis on health promotion and disease prevention."

*When to take it*: After the clinical year (3rd year or most students) and before entering residency. Most students take this exam near the end of the clinical year or early during the 4th year.

### Step 3

*What's tested*: Both basic and clinical science. The exam "assesses whether you can apply medical knowledge and understanding of biomedical and clinical science essential for the unsupervised practice of medicine, with emphasis on patient management in ambulatory settings"

*When taken*: Typically during the first year of residency.

Performing well on these exams has become a major concern for most medical students over the last few years. At a minimum, a passing score is necessary to become licensed as a doctor. But the reason that students are so concerned with performing well on board exams is because residency programs use Step 1 (and increasingly, Step2CK) scores as a key criterion for selection. On the residency director survey, Step 1 scores were second in importance only to clinical clerkship grades. The more competitive the residency, the higher the Step 1 score you'll need – and so how much effort you put toward board exams depends on your future career aspirations. If you are set on a very competitive residency such as radiation oncology, then you need to focus your efforts on exceptional board exam performance. On the other hand, if you are looking to go into a less competitive residency, such as family medicine or psychiatry, you can be less concerned with acing Step 1. On the NRMP Match website, you can find detailed charts on the average boards scores of each medical specialty.

No matter what your goals are, we're confident that our learning methods will enable you achieve them with less stress and more confidence, since you won't need to cram the way most test-takers do. But even with the superior methods we describe in this book, your effort must still be commensurate with your goal. Getting a 260 on Step 1 will require much more effort than getting a 225, and so you must make a decision about what your goal is and how much time you're willing to dedicate to this learning goal.

There is a specific body of knowledge that is tested by the various USMLE exams, as we've alluded to above. Some of that knowledge is valuable and worth retaining for life. But some of the "Step-specific" knowledge is low-yield minutiae that will have little bearing on your future career as a clinician. This is especially true of Step 1. Step 2CK is designed to be more clinically relevant, and therefore, will likely serve you better in the future, but because of its broad scope, it necessarily means you'll spend time learning things that will not show up frequently in your career.

You might find yourself saying, "Do I really need to know that mantle cell lymphoma has an 11:14 chromosomal translocation involving cyclin D1?" For Step 1, the answer is yes. For everything else in medicine? Likely not, unless you become a specialist in oncology. These facts aren't unimportant per se, but at this early stage in our careers, there are more useful and widely applicable things to focus on.

So studying for board exams means learning the specific content that is tested on the USMLE exams. You'll find the bulk of this knowledge in books like *First Aid for the USMLE Step 1*. Often this knowledge will overlap with your other goals of learning for life and learning for school, and so you can satisfy multiple goals at once (very efficient). But sometimes you will have to make dedicated efforts to acquire this narrowly focused body of knowledge, with the understanding that after you take the exam, you won't get much use from it again.

## Learning for life

Learning for life means focusing on the knowledge and skills that will be most useful to you in your practice as a physician. Depending on what you field of medicine you choose, what constitutes "learning for life" will be different. If you're going to become a surgeon, mastering anatomy is going to be more important for you than for your colleague who wants to be an endocrinologist. Likewise, future cardiologists might want to focus more on cardiac pathology rather than learning to recognize the obscure skin lesions that a dermatologist addresses.

On the other hand, some aspects of medicine are common throughout all fields. There is a core body of knowledge that nearly all physicians should know and will employ regularly. This includes physical exam skills, interviewing skills, and a basic understanding about various disease processes and treatment. We might also add certain "soft skills" such as effective communication, bedside manner, and empathy.

Learning for life also requires us to be a bit prophetic since we must envision our future careers and forecast what will be important to know in a decade or two down the line. In the last chapter of this book, we will share with you some of our best guesses about what competencies and knowledge will become increasingly important for the 21st century physician.

Our view in this book is that learning for life takes precedence over the other learning goals. That is the lens through which we make our recommendations. We prioritize learning for life because we think it pays back the most dividends for your investment of time and energy. It will likely also be the most enjoyable too, since this learning is driven by intrinsic interests and motivation rather than external carrots and sticks.

## Full Disclosure – Our approach

Whenever possible, we aim to satisfy all your learning goals simultaneously. But that's not always possible, and sometimes one goal must take precedence over others. For us, that means prioritizing learning for life. In keeping with our emphasis on long-term learning that helps you become an effective doctor, we believe that that learning for life takes precedence over learning for boards, which take precedence over learning for school.

Our experience was shaped having the luxury of going to a school whose preclinical exams are pass/fail. However, we recognize that not every school is as flexible as ours; some schools still have graded preclinical years, and so learning for school will have to take higher priority. That goal will change what materials you should learn from and how you should learn it, and as we go along, we'll offer suggestions for those whose priorities differ from ours.

## Set your goals

In the previous section, we gave you three broad goals: learning for school, learning for boards and learning for life. These goals point you toward your destination, but they don't tell you the exact steps to get where you want to go. We need to create a specific action plan for learning by breaking down our goals into discrete tasks.

# SMART Goals

A useful method for effective goal setting that has been used widely in educational settings is the **SMART** goal method. SMART is an acronym for five traits of effective goal setting:

- **S**pecific
- **M**easurable
- **A**ttainable or Actionable
- **R**esults-based
- **T**ime-related

Let's use a realistic example. In the figure below, we start with one of our broad mission goals: learning for class. This goal is laudable and worthwhile, but it's not SMART. So we need to break it down further.

First, we need our goals to be specific. So, in our case, we go from "Learn for Class" downward to increasing levels of specificity. The first level down is "Get Honors in Physiology Course." That is a SMART goal, since it's specific, measurable, attainable, results-based and time related. But now we need to define the actionable tasks that can help us achieve that goal. And so we must flesh out our SMART goals with increasingly granular tasks that will advance us toward the end we seek.

You can follow the hierarchy all the way down to the bottom level, where our goal-oriented tasks are very granular, like "Do Problem Set 2 @10 am on 2/11/15". The level of granularity at the bottom of our diagram is ultimately where you'd like to be. The more granular you make the actions that lead to your ultimate goal, the easier your learning and practice will be.

Note: Not every goal here is detailed explicitly for space's sake. We only expanded certain ones for illustration.

As you can see, the ultimate list of goals and subgoals can get large very quickly. We advise that you keep a written, visible and organized record of your goals and actions. You can use whatever medium you like – paper, text file on your computer, white board, whatever. What matters is that you have an external record of your goals and actions in

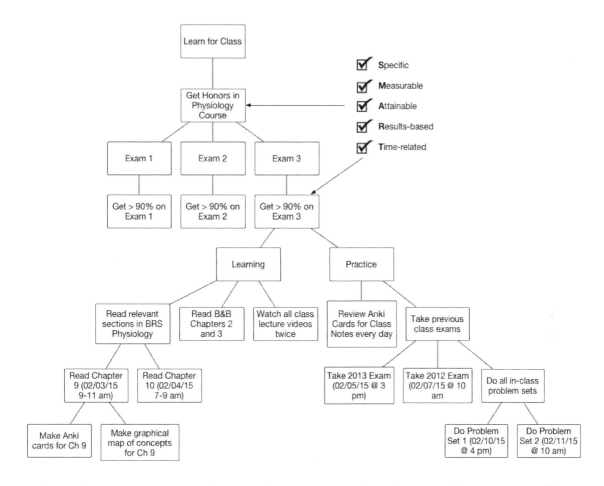

a place where you can see and review them. Using a flow diagram like ours can help you literally see how your goals align with each other, while a checklist is more useful for executing those goals.

## Scheduling with your calendar

Having established granular, goal-oriented action steps, you need to decide *when* you will do these things. Thus, we're going to make heavy use of a calendar. We ourselves use digital calendar programs like Google Calendar and Calendar.app (Mac) to help us keep track of everything. Deciding in advance when and which specific tasks you will carry helps you to avoid decision fatigue. Rather than constantly having to think about what to learn next, you have your list of tasks in front of you. And committing your learning tasks to a visible, external record can help push you to actually do them.

## Review and Re-evaluate

Even our best-laid plans need to be re-evaluated and remade periodically. Sometimes life events disrupt our plans, and sometimes our goals change with time. Thus, we recommend that you take time out every week to reevaluate and update your goals and schedule. During this time, you can take stock of the things you've done in the last week, and readjust for the coming week. But don't try to plan in detail too far out. The further ahead in time you try to plan, the less accurate you're going to be.

# Study Blocks

How long should your learning tasks be? 4 hours? 30 minutes? This may seem like an issue of personal preference, but there are actually some important guidelines for how long you should spend learning.

**Our recommendation is to work in blocks of time, creatively called study blocks, which are between 60-90 minutes of continuous work time.** After the end of a study block, take a break, do something else for a time, and then start another study block. This recommendation takes into account two critical factors: *attention* and *energy*.

We all know from personal experience that attention is a fleeting thing. Some estimates suggest that adult learners can only pay attention for 10-15 minutes before losing focus.

On the other hand, if we could only really pay attention for 15 minutes, we wouldn't have time to learn much of anything. The good news is that breaks in concentration are not permanent.

A recent study by Bunce *et al.* conducted in a college chemistry classroom found that attention follows a waxing and waning pattern during a study session, with periods of attention alternating with lapses and then recovery.[4] Lapses were few and far between at the beginning, but increased in frequency as the lecture went on. By the end of the lecture, rather than every 15 minutes, students showed lapses nearly every 2 minutes! This suggests that 60-90 minute periods are a good compromise. These blocks are long enough to let you fully wrap your head around even the most challenging material, but not so long that lapses in concentration become crippling.

The other constraint is energy. As much as we'd like to be, we humans are not machines that can just turn on and off at will. Our energy and alertness is not constant, but

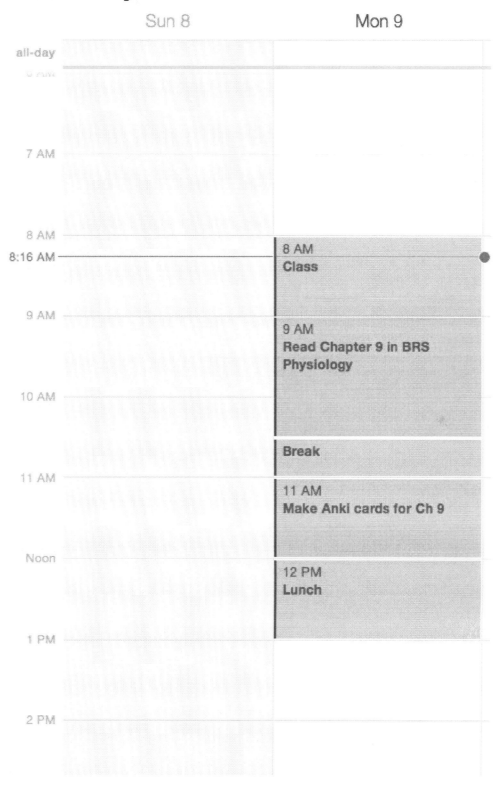

# February 2015

rather cyclical. We have periods where we feel full of energy and enthusiasm, able to conquer the world. And then we have other moments where we don't even want to move off the couch to get the remote. Ideally, we would coordinate our learning time with those periods of peak alertness and do something else during the valleys.

This idea that we should respect our physiology to maximize our productivity is the core theme of the book *The Power of Full Engagement* by author Tony Schwartz. In his book, Schwartz argues that we should adopt the practice of working intensely for 90 minutes at a time followed by a 20-30 minute break. He bases this prescription mainly on the works of chronobiologist Peretz Lavie and psychologist K. Anders Ericsson (of Deliberate Practice fame). Lavie's research demonstrated that wakefulness in humans tends to cycle with a period of roughly 90-120 minutes,[5,6] and similarly, Ericsson found that elite performers such as violinists or chess players work in intense, uninterrupted sessions that generally last between 1 and 2 hours.[7]

On the whole, we find Schwartz's 90-minute prescription to be sensible. (So much so, in fact, that we wrote much of this book in that way). However, the 90-minute figure is an average, and there is likely a lot of variation between people. The important thing is to work in sync with your own alertness rhythm by studying in sustained bursts with intervening breaks. We encourage you to experiment with different study block lengths to find the best practice for you.

If you're like most med students, this idea of taking a break is probably already making you feel dirty. It's OK. We've been there. It's deeply ingrained in medical culture to just keep working, because if you're not, somebody else is. Don't fall into this guilt trap. Respecting your physiology helps you work smarter not harder. Trying to learn medicine when you're feeling groggy or burnt out is the definition of low-yield. In those moments, you'd be better off taking a short break. Go outside, have a meal, or even take a short nap.

> "Work in sync with your own alertness rhythm by studying in sustained bursts with intervening breaks."

## Focus

We live in a time where there are more things vying for our attention than ever before. Facebook, e-mail, YouTube, Netflix, smart phones – all these things are useful, but they can also be hugely distracting when we need to focus tasks like learning.

Accordingly, we recommend that when you study, you turn off your phone. Close all potentially distracting apps on your computer: e-mail, Twitter, etc. If you don't trust yourself to not re-open these applications, install blocker apps such as Self-Control or StayFocusd for Chrome that will make it impossible for you to visit certain websites, use certain apps or open your email. And turn off the television. You may think you're learning while watching that basketball game, but you're really not. Your brain just can't do those two things at once; multi-tasking is a myth.

## Studying with others

Should you study alone or with friends? Ask yourself, "Will I be distracted if so-and-so is around?" Many med students we've talked to say that learning in groups is often not effective for them because they become too distracted by the opportunity to socialize rather than study. On the other hand, some students learn *better* with groups for a number of reasons: accountability, motivation, the ability to talk-out challenging concepts, and testing one another. The choice is yours, but just be honest with yourself.

## Where to study

Another factor that affects your focus is *where* you do your studying. Is it in the library or a coffee shop? In your home office or on your couch? Again, that's a matter of personal preference, and you should try various places to see where you find yourself most engaged and the least distracted. Both of us find that we work best with complete quiet in our respective home offices. A place like a coffee shop, with so many sights and sounds, would be sensory overload and prevent us from doing as much learning as possible. On the other hand, some of our friends find the complete silence of a library to be distracting in itself, and need the white noise of a public place to get to work.

## Sit, Stand, Walk – What kind of desk?

We learn from an early age to sit down while reading or writing, usually at a desk, sometimes on the couch or a comfortable chair if we're at home. But that's not the only option, and it may not be the best way to study, either for our health or for our learning.

In recent years, there has been a lot of talk about the dangers of sitting too much. It turns out that sitting 8 hours a day at a desk isn't great for your health. A 123,000-patient epidemiological study sponsored by the American Cancer Society found that spending 6 or more hours sitting per day was associated with higher mortality, even after controlling for exercise.[8] Several other studies have made similar findings.[9] As a result, many people have started using standing- and adjustable-height desks as a healthier way to work.

That's fine and good, but why are we talking about alternative desk setups in relation to focusing? Well, standing desks and treadmill desks may help you stay more focused and alert while working. One randomized, crossover study conducted by Dutta *et al.* used adjustable height ("sit-stand") desks in the workplace with a cohort of 28 individuals. Over the course of a 40 hour work week, they found that when the subjects used sit-stand desks, they reported feeling more energetic, less tired, less sluggish and even more calm.[10] Similarly, a study conducted by researchers from the University of Oklahoma found that subjects who used a treadmill desk had higher self-perceived 'on-task' attention. They also got 34% more questions correct on a recall task after 40 minutes of reading, and had increased EEG activity in brain regions important for memory and attentional processes.[11]

Both of us have been using adjustable-height desks throughout medical school and neither of us now wants to go back to sitting for hours on end. Like many who have switched to standing or walking, we feel much more alert and energetic while working. It's hard to get sleepy while you're standing, but much easier when you're sitting on a couch. If this interests you, don't go out and buy an expensive standing desk for $1000 or more. Search online and you'll find a number of hacks to rig a standing desk to try out.

## Task-switching

Finally, another principle is to reduce **task-switching** whenever possible. This includes going from reading to taking notes, or from watching videos to reviewing Anki cards. Whenever you switch tasks to something new, it takes some time and processing power for your brain to get oriented to the new task.[12] By sticking to one task at a time rather than flitting between several, we give ourselves more focus and study more efficiently.

# Gather the right resources

## Class, Streaming, or Self-Study?

Should you go to lecture in person, stream lectures at home, or follow the syllabus but read on your own?

This is a question a lot of students spend a lot of time first year trying to figure out, and we wish there were a single right answer. Each person has different needs and circumstances, and one size couldn't possibly fit all. What we can do, however, is provide you with a systematic way of deciding what modalities and materials to base your study efforts on.

In this section, we will briefly describe the three main learning methods in medical school. We will then discuss the major variables you should consider in deciding what sources to use. We don't expect any single resource to monopolize your time; rather, we will equip you with the principles to decide, in each given situation, what resources will best help you reach your goals.

There are three major categories of resources that will be available to you in medical school. They are:

1. **Attending lectures in person**. This is the same modality that you've used for your decade-plus schooling career, and many of the same advantages and disadvantages. You get face time with the professors, and some students find that being there in person forces them to stay attentive. At the same time, the quality of lectures in medical school can be variable, and in-person attendance lacks some of the nifty features of video streaming.

2. **Video streaming lectures**: This is a new technology that most medical schools have implemented. Each day, the lectures are recorded and put online for you to stream. This has several advantages. It is more convenient; you can study in whatever environment works best for you – in your apartment, with friends in the library, or at a local coffee shop. It is flexible with respect to time, so that you can watch lectures whenever you are most alert, or run an errand in the middle of class time.

   Most interestingly, though, video streaming lets you control the pace of the lecture. If the lecturer talks slowly or is covering material you are already familiar with, you can zip through it at 2x normal play speed. If he's explaining a tricky point, you can slow it down to 1x and even go back to hear the explanation a second time. You can also skip poorly presented lectures altogether. This time savings and flexibility make streaming very attractive to learners like us.

3. **Learning on your own:** This is by far the broadest category. There is a wide variety of material you can use to learn medicine on your own, from review books to professional video series like the Pathoma lectures. You can use your course syllabus to guide your reading, but otherwise rely primarily on outside texts and video for your learning.

It would be nice if you could just depend on your medical school to feed you all the information you need in the best package, but that's not the case. It's on you to find the best learning resources for the subject you're learning, and tailor your reading list to your needs. Below, we'll give you some thoughts on the matter.

## Modality

There are two major channels through which information can reach our brains: our eyes (visual) and our ears (auditory). Both are important for learning, but our brains show a definite preference for the visual channel – which is why we say "a picture is worth a thousand words."

> "Our brains show a definite preference for the visual channel – which is why we say 'a picture is worth a thousand words.'"

Our operating principle is that we should aim to engage both channels simultaneously, and that we should avoid cognitive overload by having the auditory and visual channels perform, complementary, non-overlapping roles.[13] A lecture video in which an instructor narrates a slide that has just a figure on it, without a lot of adjoining text, is an example of dual-channel learning where the visuals and audio work together, rather than overwhelming the learner.

Put it all together, and we have the following hierarchy: **Videos > Text > Audio only.**

Now, there is certainly an element of personal preference involved. We've heard things such as "I get so bored when I read a textbook" or "Lectures put me to sleep." And even the same person might even have variable preferences depending on mood, context, energy level, or time of day. So take our hierarchy as a guideline, but pay attention to your preferences and go with what you're most likely to use. If you hate reading textbooks, don't make textbooks your primary source for learning. Likewise, if your preferred way of learning is video, look for the best video sources you can find.

## Learning at the right level

Another major factor we must consider is **level of detail.** Knowledge can be represented on a spectrum of detail, from general to specific. How much detail you need depends on your learning goals and also your level of prior knowledge.

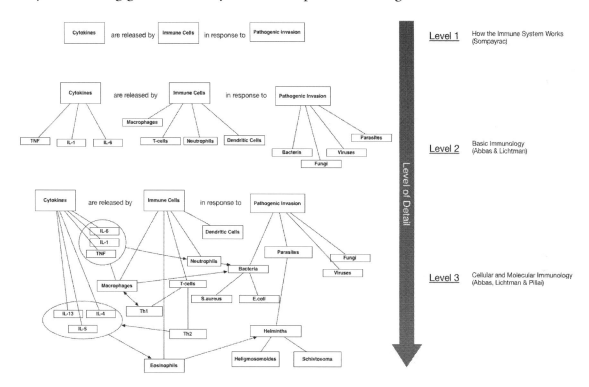

To illustrate, let's look at this figure. At the top, we have a factual statement about immunology: "Cytokines are released by immune cells in response to pathogenic invasion." This statement is at a low level of detail, giving a "big picture" view of an idea. Its major components – "cytokines," "immune cells" and "pathogenic invasion" – are general terms representing broad classes or concepts. In effect, these general terms hide many details under the hood, allowing you to focus on the substance of the idea and the major relationships among the components – "are released by" and "in response to." Let's say that this piece of knowledge lies at Level 1 on our scale.

We can expand this statement by adding some specifics, represented in Level 2 of the figure. There are dozens of cytokines, but let's expand that term and add some of the major ones: TNF, IL-1 and IL-6. These are important members of the class "cytokine," though we omitted many others. And how about immune cells? There are several, so let's flesh out some of the main ones here. And finally, let's flesh out the several types of pathogens that can invade and infect the body, including bacteria, fungi, viruses and parasites. What we've done here is peered under the hood a little to see some of the specific details encompassed by the level 1 statement. Each level is an additional layer of detail added on top of the core idea.

Of course, there is still much more detail we could add to our core statement. Moving down to Level 3, we've added yet further specific details on top of the core. There are more cytokines, and we've indicated that they are released by certain types of immune cells in response to specific kinds of invaders. Bacteria elicit different cytokine release patterns than do helminths, a type of parasite, and we've represented that here. There is still a ton we've left out, but we'll stop here. The point is clear: knowledge can be represented with varying levels of detail, with a central core idea and then layers of specifics added on top.

## From forest to leaves

Let's say you've never taken an immunology course before, so you have little prior knowledge about the subject. At what level would you begin your learning? Would you pick a reference textbook (Level 3) and just start plowing away? Or would you start with an introductory text that operates at Levels 1-2?

Being the high achieving medical student that you are, you might be inclined to say Level 3. "I'm going right for nitty gritty. I don't need training wheels." This strategy will not get you very far, however. Why? Because when you jump straight to detailed knowledge, all that information *has little meaning to you*. Recall from *Brain Science* that a major factor determining the effective storage of new information is how much prior knowledge we have. Learning is easiest when we can connect new information to prior knowledge. The problem with starting deep in the weeds of Level 3 is that as a beginner, you just get lost in a morass of minute details that are hard to make sense of, leaving your brain overwhelmed.

Moreover, you'll miss the forest for the trees. Caught up in details, you won't notice the core propositions, such as "Cytokines are released by immune cells in response to pathogenic invaders." General principles like these are not always obvious, especially to the novice. Good textbooks and good teachers spell it out for you, but many sources do not, leaving you to formulate the "big picture" view yourself.

The right approach, then, is to move sequentially from lower levels of detail to higher levels of detail, building your knowledge successively, layer by layer. Learning this way will enable you to absorb and understand far more knowledge than if you dive right into the deep end

Learning in this sequential manner also helps you learn strategically. Most of us will develop expertise in particular specialties, where our knowledge will be rich and deep. For those things, we would want to eventually acquire highly detailed, Level 3 knowledge.

> "Move sequentially from lower levels of detail to higher levels of detail."

For everything else, the big picture view is sufficient, since you can always look up the details from an external reference. But in order to even know what to look for, you need to have some knowledge to steer your search efforts. That is what Level 1 and 2 knowledge can do for you. It's just enough for you to see important relationships, and with these general insights in mind, you can then go to a reference source to find the relevant details when you need them.

How do you know what level a resource is? For common subjects, textbook authors have done a lot of the work for us. They, too, know that novices and experts need different levels of detail, and are careful to target their books at a specific audience. Indeed, sometimes the same book will be reformatted to serve those different audiences. Examples include the Robbins Pathology family ("little, medium and big Robbins") and the Harrison's family (pocket Harrison's, big Harrison's).

In our figure, we've actually included a real progression that we think illustrates the levels of knowledge for learning immunology. At level 1 is an excellent, big picture primer called *How the Immune System Works*. If you were just starting out, you should definitely read this first to give you the broad elements and relationships in immunology. Then, to get more detail, you would advance to *Basic Immunology* by Abbas and Lichtman. If you wanted still further detail, you could progress to *Cellular and Molecular Immunology*, also by Abbas and Lichtman.

By learning in this sequential manner, you would absorb, understand and remember the maximum amount of information. Try to jump in with *Cellular and Molecular Immunology* and you will likely be frustrated. Indeed, med students often complain that a subject like immunology is challenging and complicated – and one reason is that professors, who are experts, sometimes assign Level 3 resources right from the outset, bombarding and overwhelming their students. Smart students will trust their own judgment and choose introductory books to start off with instead.

We recognize that figuring out resource's level of detail is challenging in the beginning, when the whole subject is new. To help you out, in the *Implementation* section, we've gone through some of the major texts in each topic and described their usefulness and level of detail.

## Bringing it together

Between sensory modality, personal preference, and levels of organization, rarely will one resource cover all the criteria well enough. So, it is best to use multiple resources to compensate for the deficiencies in each individual source.

Use the provided principles to think about how to use each resource, but ultimately you will have to experience each modality for yourself to make informed decisions. How good are your school's lecturers? How much do you like setting your own pace with streaming video? You need to experience these for yourself. For this reason, in the *Implementation* section, we recommend that you use the first few weeks of med school to experiment with different learning methods and seeing how they feel to you. Try going to lecture, try streaming. Funny as it may sound, a trial of skipping class might be the key to a good grade!

## Prime your learning

One curious insight that is emerging from the cognitive psychology research is that testing yourself on to-be-learned material *before* you acquire that material can enhance your ability to store and retrieve that information.[29-31] The insight here is that asking yourself questions about the things you're about to learn can help to prime uptake and retention of that material. Practically, this means that we should try to ask ourselves some questions before we get reading or watching.

"But what about if I don't know anything about a topic?" you may be asking yourself. Perhaps you're about to read about renal physiology for the first time, and GFR or podocytes mean nothing to you. How could you answer questions about this correctly? In instances like this, you'll almost certainly be without the correct answer, but even still, the act of trying to produce an answer to a question will still yield benefits during your later acquisition by focusing your mind toward specific pieces of information in your source material. So where do pre-test questions come from? We have a couple of sources. If you have access to pre-made SRS content that is relevant to the material you'll be learning, then you can easily use your SRS cards to test yourself before you learn. The key here is that your cards match the content you're about to learn. So, for example, if you are about to read the Fungi chapter from *Clinical Microbiology Made Ridiculously Simple* and you have SRS cards that closely match that chapter (perhaps a deck made by upperclassmen), testing yourself on these cards before reading would be expected to enhance your retention of the to-be-learned material.

We don't always have access to such well-made and well-matched SRS cards in advance of learning and making our own. Thus, an alternative place we can look for pre-test questions is the end of a chapter. Most good textbooks have end-of-chapter questions. We can also create our own by turning chapter headings/subheadings as well as bolded terms into questions. For example, if you're reading about hematology, and there is a chapter subheading on 'Clotting Cascade', you can turn this into a question by asking yourself "What is the clotting cascade and what do I already know about it?" Finally, if you're operating at the detail level 2 or 3, you might try some practice questions before you read or watch a video.

## Think and organize

In *Brain Science*, we discussed how thinking deeply about something improves your ability to remember that information, and how well organized knowledge is easier to retrieve than disordered knowledge. We spoke broadly about these ideas in the previous sections, but now we need to get specific. In this section, we will provide evidence-based practices that will help you to think about and organize your learning in the most effective ways.

# The value of frameworks

One simple and effective tool for helping us to organize our knowledge is the **framework.** Simply put, a framework is a pre-determined structure for organizing knowledge. A good framework gives us mental slots where we can easily place new information.

To make this more concrete, let's talk about a specific example of a framework in anatomy: the muscle table. When you learn about each muscle, you think of the following aspects:

- Origin
- Insertion
- Function
- Nerves
- Blood Supply

The nice thing about this framework is that it provides a unified way to approach each new muscle you learn. Every muscle has these components. When you get new information about a muscle, you can use this structure to place facts into their appropriate bins. Not thinking with this framework in mind makes it harder to keep all the facts together, and therefore, harder to retrieve later on.

Developing a framework takes both time and knowledge of the subject matter. That's why we have also provided frameworks for each medical section in the *Implementation* section of this book. We've spent time thinking about how best to organize information for the various subjects that one encounters in medicine. You can use the frameworks we provide as a starting point. As you go through your studies, you can modify and customize them to suit your needs.

At some point, however, you'll need to develop frameworks on your own. So how do you come up with a framework? And how do you know what framework to use before you even start studying? There are several options.

The easiest way is to rely on the expertise of your learning resources. The people who make the best textbooks, review books, and videos have often thought a lot about how to optimally organize the content. Therefore, you should use the structure of the learning resource to help you create your own framework. Look at the table of contents. See how the book is organized. Look at the chapter headings and subheadings. The tables and figures within chapters also provide important guidance about how to frame the content.

Sometimes you can also use your prior knowledge about a subject: Ask yourself what you already know, and see whether a logical organizational scheme is apparent. In the anatomy example, it would be logical to assume that when learning about blood vessels, for example, you should attend to what other blood vessels they are connected to, and what tissues and organs they supply blood to.

Finally, you can ask an expert. Ask your teachers or your classmates how they organize the knowledge that you are learning. This can be very valuable, but keep in mind that sometimes experts forget what it was like to be a novice. Therefore, the way they organize information is not always appropriate for new learners. So it is worth asking but do take their organization scheme with a grain of salt.

## Self-Explanation

You've no doubt had the experience of sitting for hours with a book, and realizing at the end that you barely remember what you've read. We want to help you avoid that scenario. So what tools do we have at our disposal?

One effective method with ample support is called **self-explanation.** Formally, self-explanation is "explaining how new information is related to known information or explaining steps taken during problem solving.[14] Self-explanation has been demonstrated to be effective in a variety of educational contexts, including medicine.

For example, a recent study by Larsen and colleagues conducted at the Washington University in St. Louis Medical School found that students who used self-explanation in conjunction with their studying performed better on a 6-month follow-up test than students who just studied.[15]

For factual knowledge, which most of what we deal with in medicine, you can use the following templates for self-explanation, adapted from Chi *et al.*[16] and Hausmann *et al.*[17]:

1. What new information have you seen?
2. How does this information relate to what you already know?
3. Does this new information give you insight into your understanding of this subject?
4. Does this information raise a question in your mind?

When you're learning from a 'worked problem', a different set of prompts are appropriate (Adapted from Hausmann *et al.* and Conati *et al.*[17,18])

1.  What principle is being applied in this step?
2.  This choice is correct because…
3.  What is the justification for this step? Why is it correct?
4.  What law, definition or rule allows one to draw that conclusion?

Self-explanation can be used in several steps of the learning process. The first place is during the Acquire step. Self-explanation, by its nature, is an active learning technique since it forces you to generate answers and make connections among knowledge, and can help you learn new material more effectively.

Another time to use self-explanation is when you're doing practice problems, such as practice problems from USMLE World. Rather than just reading the explanation and accepting it on face value, you could explain to yourself why the correct answer is correct. For such scenarios, you could use the second set of prompts above, which were designed for worked problems.

While self-explanation is effective, it does take time. When is it most worth taking the time? For factual knowledge, self-explanation is most effective when you have prior *misconceptions* or conflicting target knowledge. So you should use these prompts when you've learned something that is confusing or unclear to you or is in conflict with your prior knowledge.[19] For problem solving, on the other hand, self-explanation is most effective when you have *little to no* prior knowledge of the concepts or procedures. So you should use the problem-solving prompts when you are doing practice problems that correspond to topics you're less familiar with.

## Graphical and Textual Organizers

Another useful way to help you build connected knowledge is to represent what you know in graphical form. As we discussed in *Brain Science,* our minds have a clear preference for things that are visual. Remembering an image, such as a biochemical pathway or anatomical diagram, can help you retrieve a lot of information that you might have a hard time doing otherwise. So we think it's valuable to try to visualize your knowledge and make explicit connections in a way you can see.

This needn't be fancy. You can represent your knowledge with something as simple as a rough concept map or Venn diagram. What we do recommend, though, is that you first attempt to make your graphic *from memory*, without referring to source material. By making your graphic from memory, you're actually practicing retrieval at the same time, which enhances your memory of the knowledge you recall.

However, once you have made your attempt at producing a graphic, then you *should* refer to the source material to make sure that you have correctly represented the information. This immediate feedback is critical because it will help you to correct misconceptions early. Otherwise you may internalize the wrong information, based on your misunderstanding of the material.

While making your graphical organizer, you should focus not just on the facts or ideas but also on their relationships. This forces you to create relationships between ideas, which is a key part of understanding any topic in depth.

# Chapter 10:
# Acquire

Now that we've covered the preliminaries, and you have prepared yourself to absorb new information, it is time to actually get down to it. In the preclinical years, the major sources of information are texts (e.g. textbooks, articles, class notes, etc.) and videos. Acquiring from each of these sources requires a slightly different approach, and we're going to give you a step-by-step guide on how to learn from these sources most effectively.

## Acquiring from texts

Given that you're reading this book right now, it might seem silly at first that we would have a whole section instructing you on how to acquire from texts. If you can read words on a page, that's all there is to it, right? Not exactly. We can all run our eyes over pages of text, which is reading. But as we know from common experience, two people can read the same text and end up with very different knowledge outcomes. Why is that? Well, a lot of it has to do with the mental processes that one uses while engaging with a text. As we discussed in depth in the Brain Science section, even something simple like reading some words on a page is really a complex orchestration of many mental activities, and if we want to maximize what and how much of those words on a page make it into our minds for the long-term, there are things we need to work on.

And so, in this section, we're going to instruct you on how to read more effectively, so as to maximize the likelihood of acquiring the right pieces of information and remembering them for the long-term.

# Reading rules

1. Read linearly through a text one paragraph at a time. Also, examine text figures and tables in sequence.

2. After completing each paragraph or figure, stop to highlight anything that you will want to capture and extract later on. Use the Aids to Acquisition section (described below) to help you decide what is worth highlighting. Do not highlight while reading a paragraph, as this will interrupt your flow. Wait until the end, and then go back.

3. Before moving on to the next paragraph or figure, pause briefly to reflect on what you just read. In particular, think about the content in light of your framework and the advance organizers you used in your preparation.

4. If something doesn't make sense, either re-read the text or use a reference source to clarify an unknown.

5. Move on and repeat until done with your reading.

Let's discuss these rules further. The first needs little explanation – texts are usually written to be read in a linear fashion, with figures and tables presented in a useful sequence, there's little to be gained by jumping around.

Rule #2 is where things get interesting. Part of the acquisition process is to mark certain pieces of information for later capture and extraction into our SRS. The question though is when should you do this – while you are reading or after? Our recommendation is to read a paragraph in full, without interruption. When finished, then you can go back to the text and highlight the important pieces. It's a minimally intrusive practice that doesn't take your focus away from the ideas on the page. Above all, the important thing is to capture important nuggets of information without getting distracted by the note-taking process itself. Moreover, you get a better sense of what's worth marking after reading the complete package of ideas in a paragraph, rather than marking while reading. Hopefully in this way, you avoid the problem of a 'jaundiced textbook' where everything is highlighted.

> "The important thing is to capture important nuggets of information without getting distracted by the note-taking process itself."

Rule #3 is also probably something new to you. Most students read a paragraph and then plow on to the next one without pausing. Why should you pause? There are several reasons. First, the end of a paragraph is a natural checkpoint for you to ensure that you have registered the ideas in the text you just read and that it makes sense to you. There is no point in moving on if the last paragraph, upon which subsequent ideas will build, doesn't click for you. Second, the end-of-paragraph pause provides an excellent and much needed place for you to impart some organization and structure to the ideas you just read. What does that look like specifically? This is where having a framework comes in handy. Let's look at a section from Robbins Pathology to illustrate how the framework can be used.

> "Almost all cases of acute mastitis occur during the first month of breastfeeding. *(Epidemiology)* During this time the breast is vulnerable to bacterial infection because of the development of cracks and fissures in the nipples. From this portal of entry, *Staphylococcus aureus* or, less commonly, streptococci invade the breast tissue. *(Etiology)* The breast is erythematous and painful, and fever is often present. At the outset only one duct system or sector of the breast is involved. *(Clinical Signs/Symptoms)* If not treated the infection may spread to the entire breast. *(Complications)* Most cases of lactational mastitis are easily treated with appropriate antibiotics and continued expression of milk from the breast. Rarely, surgical drainage is required. *(Treatment)*" From: *Robbins Pathologic Basis of Disease* (12 ed.)

This paragraph is discussing acute mastitis, which is an infectious disease of the breast. For diseases, we use the familiar and useful disease framework, which relates each disease to its epidemiology, time course, etiology, pathogenesis, sign and symptoms, and treatment. (We'll discuss the Disease framework in the *Implementation* section.) Our little block of prose has facts pertaining to each of these mental "slots" in our disease framework, but there's no indication of that. It is left to the reader to mentally sort out the different pieces of information into their respective slots in the framework. Pausing after reading a paragraph like this gives us the first opportunity to plug in the new information into our familiar mental framework that helps us to organize this information as it enters our working and long-term memory, which will help with remembering later on.

In addition to organizing, you can also check yourself for understanding. Let's say that you didn't know that *S. aureus* and *Streptococci* were types of bacteria because you were slacking off during microbiology. The paragraph then wouldn't be entirely clear because you didn't know that the causes of acute mastitis are infectious bacterial pathogens. So, at this point, you might be prompted to quickly Google *S. aureus* or *Streptococci* before moving onward in your reading. This is Rule # 4, which also helps consolidate your knowledge.

At this point, you might object that pausing will slow you down too much in your reading. It's true, taking a pause will reduce the pace at which you read, but it will also increase the amount of information that you successfully acquire. What is the point of reading rapidly if little of it sticks? We think the minor cost of a slower pace of reading is greatly outweighed by the gains you'll make in effective storage and subsequent retrieval the newly learned material.

# Aids to acquisition in texts

As we discussed earlier, one of the major challenges of learning is filtering the important from the less important, the high-yield from the low-yield. One of the benefits of acquiring from high-quality texts, such as the textbooks we frequently encounter in medical school, is that a team of experts and editors spent a lot of time and energy making these choices in writing the text. Moreover, any good textbook will be crafted so as to make it as clear and easy as possible for the reader to absorb the information. The key for you, as the learner, is to recognize these aids and use them to help you acquire. Many learners don't fully utilize these helpful features, and miss out on the benefits they bring to learning.

## Headings and subheadings

Headings and subheadings are the big signposts in a text that tell you broadly what is to come. More importantly, they indicate the major conceptual elements of the subject matter at hand. You can learn a lot just from looking at the chapter outline in the table of contents or at the beginning of a chapter. When the author drafted an outline of the textbook, he likely started with the headings and subheadings, which reflect the way that the author thinks about and mentally organizes that material. Let this guide the way you acquire and organize that information in your head as it goes in.

## Topic sentences

Topic sentences are usually the first sentence in a paragraph. This sentence sets the main idea of a paragraph and indicates to the read what is to come in the following sentences in that paragraph. More times than not, the topic sentence is a general statement that is then fleshed out by specific details in the body text of a paragraph. By putting the topic sentence front and center, the author is saying to you "Look here. This is what I want you to know." You should use this to your advantage.

One book that truly exemplifies the use of strong topic sentences *is Cellular and Molecular Immunology* by Abbas, Lichtman and Pillai. This is one of the best immunology textbooks around, in our opinion, and one major reason is its clarity, which is aided by the use of sharp and prominent topic sentences. Indeed, in this text, the topic sentences are made bold and italic, to emphasize even more to the reader to "LOOK HERE!!" For example, in the chapter on innate immunity, one paragraph begins with the following:

> **"The two major types of responses of the innate immune system that protect against microbes are inflammation and antiviral defense.** Inflammation is the process by which leukocytes and circulating plasma proteins..."

The paragraph goes on then to elaborate on the details of inflammation and antiviral defense. Those details help illustrate the main point, but they aren't the main point; the topic sentence is. Use this feature to your advantage. This is a freebie when it comes to filtering. The author is telling you what he/she thinks you should know.

## Bolded Keywords or Terms

Another aid in figuring out what to look for is bolded keywords. Keywords are made bold in a text to emphasize their importance, so you should heed this signal. The emphasis is even more patent here than with topic sentences. The author is telling you that the text in bold is essential. In addition, bolded keywords are usually accompanied by a definition, which is easy fodder for SRS apps. As a general rule, if something is a bolded, you should pay attention, and expect to capture and extract this information later on.

## Figures and Tables

Figures and tables also indicate that important information lies there. Figures and tables take time and effort to make, and so authors usually only use them for the most essential ideas and concepts. Moreover, figures are often included to represent complex relationships that are difficult to articulate in words but that become clear when made visual. Accordingly, you should take notice of all the figures in a good textbook and use them to point out the important ideas and relationships among those ideas.

## End-of-chapter summaries and terms

Well-crafted, professional textbooks will often include an end-of-chapter summary of the important ideas as well as a glossary of key terms. An excellent example of such a text is *Essential Cell Biology* by Alberts *et al*. At the end of every chapter, there are several summary statements related to the chapter content as well as a glossary of the important, bolded terms.

These useful aids add a lot of value. The author has done so much of the heavy lifting for you at the end, using their knowledge and perspective to provide succinct statements that capture the essential ideas and definitions. If a summary and glossary is included in a source, use them too. All this information may even be good enough to go right into your SRS, without any further transformation.

Moreover, you should use these summaries and terms to gauge your understanding. If a statement or term is entirely foreign to you or you don't understand, that's a sign you should go back to the text and make sure your grasp that material.

## Reflecting with self-explanation

Earlier we introduced the technique of self-explanation to enhance your understanding. It's a powerful tool, but it also takes some time, and so we recommend using it selectively. Rather than applying it after every paragraph, we suggest using self-explanation in chapter sections or subsections, which usually correspond to a single topic or idea. For example, if you're reading about Pathology, the chapter text is likely broken down by diseases or overarching ideas. Applying self-explanation prompts quickly at the end of such sections is good practice. You'll need to use your judgment based on the amount of time you have and how well you already know the material, but this is our base recommendation.

## Extract to SRS

After you've finished your reading, it is time to take the highlights and annotations you made and move them into your SRS. For detailed guidance on how to render your highlights into high quality cards using refer to our discussion of how to make good cards in the *Spaced Repetition Software* section.

Depending on your goals, you may choose to extract all of your markings/annotations or only a portion of them. You should commit only those bits of information that you really need for long-term memory. Cram-and-forget material can go into a separate note sheet or Word document.

# Acquiring from video

Increasingly, educational resources are being digitized in the form of video recordings. For several years now, medical students have been electing to stay at home and watch recorded lectures on their computer (streaming), rather than show up for class. The rest of the world is catching up to med students in the form of massive open online courses (MOOCs). It's an incredible time to be a learner, since so many high quality learning tools are coming to the fore, accessible to just about everyone.

Video learning has several advantages. The major benefit is the ability to watch lectures at your own pace and at your leisure. If something is poorly explained, you can stop, go back, and watch again. If you already know what is being discussed, you can skip past that part. You can also increase the speed to 1.5x or 2x, and pick up the pace. Some students get so used to listening at this speed that live lectures seem slow by comparison!

We also noted earlier that combining audio and visual streams has been shown to be more memorable than either audio or video alone. So a well-made video where someone is narrating (audio) over an explanatory figure (visual) is ideal. You get the benefit of having two sensory streams working at the same time, enhancing encoding and hopefully, later retrieval.

However, for all of its benefits, video has creates new challenges for acquiring. First, videos often do not come with accompanying text, which makes it harder for you to make flashcards later on. If a video does not have text, you'll need to take notes while watching the video, which amounts to more work, a slower pace, and a breaking of focus. At many medical schools, the lecturer often gives out lecture slides that correspond to the video. This can help, but are not always a great substitute for a well-organized text. One strategy that may help is to read along with a text of your own, and use it as a reference while you watch the video. This might be a textbook that you know the lecturer relies on heavily, or it might be *First Aid,* which can guide you to which topics are most boards-worthy.

Second, unless they're professionally crafted, videos do not have much internal organization or aids to acquisition, as good textbooks often do. Thus, if you want to go to a particular piece of information, you need to know the exact time point at which the narrator in the video says or shows something. Often, you don't know when that is, so you need to scroll through little by little, which is inefficient and frustrating. This situation may improve in the future, since the trend seems to be towards shorter videos, each dealing with a single discrete topic, which makes for easier organization. But for the time being, many medical schools just record a 50 minute lectures leaving you to navigate through them.

Lastly, there is the issue of quality. Unlike a professional textbook, which goes through many rounds of editing and revision, video lectures are usually given once, with little or no editing. Accordingly, we find that many videos lack coherence and comprehensiveness, which requires the learner still to supplement his learning with texts. Some professionally crafted videos, like those from Pathoma, are an exception to the rule, but overall, the average video is just not as well made as the average textbook.

Despite all of these challenges, videos are still an excellent medium for acquiring new information. And for many students, video is their preferred way to learn. Thus, we will now describe how to acquire from videos, paying attention to the challenges we noted above.

## Video with accompanying textbook

The best scenario is when you are acquiring from a video series that has an accompanying text that closely follows the content of the video. The steps for acquiring from this kind of video are the following:

1. Have the accompanying text open at the part that corresponds to the video you are watching. For example, if you are watching a video entitled "Hemolytic Anemia" then you should open the book to the "Hemolytic Anemia" section.

2. Begin to watch the video, focusing on the narration and visuals. Give most of your attention to the screen, and not the accompanying text. Do not highlight or mark up your book while watching, since this is a distraction and will make it harder to absorb. Just watch the video.

3. After each conceptual section (akin to a paragraph or chapter subsection), pause the video. Go to the accompanying text and make highlights and annotations for things that you will want to convert into flashcards later on. Also, use this opportunity to think about what you just heard, making sure that everything makes sense. Think about the new information through the lens of your framework, organizing it in a way that makes sense to you.

4. Continue to the next section of the video, repeating the above steps each time.

5. Feed the information into Anki or your other spaced repetition system.

If your lecture doesn't come with notes, you should still give most of your attention to the screen, but you'll need to take notes at the same time as watching. This is not ideal, since it pulls your attention from the video content, and depending on the speed of your writing/typing, you may miss something important. To make matters more difficult, you will also need to exercise judgment as to what is worthy of writing down and what is not. That's an additional cognitive task that makes acquiring in this way more challenging. Because you need to do so many things at once, we recommend watching videos at 1x speed only in this circumstance.

Some other considerations for watching videos:

## Speed

We know that many students like to increase the speed of a video playback to save time. Depending on the natural talking speed of the lecturer, this may or may not be appropriate. If you can follow everything that is said at 1.5x or 2x speed, go for it. Just make sure that you are actually following. There is no benefit in saving a little time if you need to go back and re-watch because you didn't follow what was said in the video.

## Pause points

Above, we suggest pausing after each "conceptual section". But what does that mean? In a text, that is well defined by the natural units of text – paragraphs. However, in videos, it is not entirely clear. You will need to use your judgment. Usually, each slide is used for a different idea component, and so as a rule of thumb, you may want to pause briefly after each slide. Also, a good presenter will usually signal a transition between topics in his narration, with something like "Ok, so now let's talk about…" or "Moving on…". Use these verbal cues to guide your choice of pause points.

# Chapter 11:
## Review – Keeping It In Your Head

After we've filled our heads with hard-earned knowledge, we need to work to keep it there. That's what **Review** is for. For us, reviewing is active, not passive; it's an opportunity to practice *retrieval* of knowledge from memory, taking advantage of the testing and spacing effects. We separate out review into two steps; the **initial review** that occurs within hours after learning something, and the **maintenance reviews** that are an ongoing effort to strengthen your memory. Our trusty tool Anki plays a starring role in helping us organize and manage our review efforts.

## Initial Review

The initial review is the first review after exposure to new material. Its purpose is to retard some of the rapid forgetting that happens within the early hours after learning. This review also provides early feedback to help fill in holes and correct misunderstandings while your memory of learning the material is still fresh.

For example, imagine that you just finished learning about fungal diseases and you made some new SR cards on Anki. You could review the cards immediately afterwards, but because you literally just finished learning these facts, your initial learning will make retrieval too easy.

According to the principle of desirable difficulties, activities requiring greater mental effort are associated with greater retention.[20,21] So you want to review in such a way that recall is difficult but not impossible. Doing your initial review too far away from the time of learning will result in little to no retrieval, and too close to the time of learning will result in nearly perfect recall. Ideally, you'd like to be somewhere in between these extremes.

A useful analogy is lifting weights at the gym. Lifting very light weights may make you feel like you're doing a lot of exercise, but your strength gains will be minimal. Try to lift a weight that is too heavy for you, and you'll also get no benefit since you can't even get it off the ground. But lifting a weight that is intermediate, heavy enough to make you exert effort, but not so much that it's impossible for you, will bring you the most gains. This last scenario is what we want to apply to our retrieval practice (reviewing).

As a middle ground, we recommend that you do your first review between 30 minutes and 24 hours after studying new things. For example, you might finish your learning of new material in the afternoon on a given day. Then the next morning, do your initial reviews.

# Maintenance review

The maintenance review is for, well, maintenance. Even after an initial review, that newly acquired knowledge still has a pretty short half-life, and it must retrieved again and again in order to make the memory durable. And that goes for everything you learn, not just the new stuff.

> "We recommend that you do your first review between 30 minutes and 24 hours after studying new things."

Fortunately, SRS apps like Anki put your maintenance reviews on autopilot, so all you need to do is keep up with your reviews and trust the algorithm. That said, holding onto the massive amounts of medical knowledge you've acquired still takes daily work. Every day, Anki's spaced repetition algorithm will present the cards that need to be reviewed. This review is absolutely essential. Without it, you'll surely miss out on the benefits of Anki and our learning system.

Unlike the initial review, maintenance review doesn't have a fixed time. You can do your daily maintenance review whenever you have time during the day. All that matters is that it gets done. Anki makes it easy, since it can be used on all mobile platforms, on your desktop or the web.

One of the great advantages of Anki is its mobility. With the AnkiMobile app, you can study anywhere, anytime, and take advantage of time that might otherwise be wasted. For example, when you're doing the ten-minute walk from the parking lot to the lecture hall, that's an excellent time to do some reviews. Waiting in line in the cafeteria is another prime opportunity. Some people like to block out a chunk of time and do all their cards at once, which can be quite efficient during the preclinical year. In the clinical year, when big blocks of time are rare, the ability to do little review sprints distributed throughout the day to take advantage of pockets of free time is invaluable.

There is also some evidence that taking 'pastoral' breaks – getting outside – can boost attention and diminish mental fatigue.[22] We've both taken this to heart and spent some time in our preclinical years studying outside or taking walks while we studied – another benefit of Anki's mobility.

# Best practices for reviewing

To get the most benefit from your reviews, it is important to be in the right frame of mind. You should be focused and engaged in the review process. Don't try to watch television, talk to a friend on Facebook and do your reviews at the same time. Focus on the review.

When a card prompts you, try to come up with answer as quickly as you can. You might even use the time-to-answer as a measure of the difficulty of the card. And if you get the answer incorrect, don't just move on. Think about why you got the question wrong. Similarly, when you see the card again and you answer correctly, really stop and think about why the answer you're giving is correct. Remember that memory is the residue of thought. If you don't think about the answers you give, you'll likely not form strong memories, and will get the question wrong again at a later time. If you find yourself getting the same question incorrect time and again, it's almost certainly because you haven't actually thought about the answer you're giving. (Anki calls these cards "leeches" and flags them automatically.) You get it right in the short term because you recognize the question and know the answer, but it doesn't

> *"If you find yourself getting the same question incorrect time and again, it's almost certainly because you haven't actually thought about the answer you're giving."*

mean much to you. In order to break this cycle, you need to think about the question and answer and try to give it some meaning, to fit it into your mental network of knowledge.

# Managing your review loads

One of the common complaints we hear about Anki from our classmates is that it takes a lot of time. It's true; in the short-term, making cards and keeping up with daily maintenance reviews take a serious effort, more so than if you just did the usual cramming approach. But over the long-term, Anki is a huge time *saver* since you don't need to go back and relearn tons of material that you forgot. When we came into medical school, a lot of well-meaning upperclassmen "reassured" us that we shouldn't worry about long-term retention, since we'd have to relearn everything in a few years once we're on the wards anyway. Anki removes that burden, and so we promise your extra upfront effort with Anki will pay back big dividends later on.

Nevertheless, the short-term burden of Anki is real, and we need to talk about how to manage it. An all too common scenario is where an enthusiastic medical student finds out about Anki's effectiveness, makes hundreds of cards, does them all in a day, and then is swamped with a mountain of reviews a couple of days later. We want to help you avoid these situations, so here are some guidelines to help you:

1. Don't do more than 100 new/cards per day in your initial reviews
2. Look at your card forecasts (Anki stats). If big review days are coming up, try to put off doing new cards in the preceding day or two.
3. Spread out your maintenance review into multiple shorter sessions
4. If you do get bombed with a lot of cards, it's not the end of the world if you spread it out across a couple of days. You can use the 'review' setting to limit the number you see, so that you don't get demoralized

Finally, know that the review burden *does* lessen with time. The intervals get longer, and the cards get staggered, and so you have fewer reviews per day. Over time, they will reduce to almost nothing.

# Chapter 12:
## Apply – Putting Your Learning To Work

And now the fun part. The purpose of the preceding steps – Acquire and Review – is to set us up to do something useful with the knowledge you gained. Whether in doing practice questions, working on projects, or taking care of real patients, Apply encompasses everything you want to do with the knowledge you've accumulated.

In this section, we will discuss the major principles involved in putting knowledge into practice. We'll describe some of the many different ways that you will apply your knowledge in medical contexts and give specific steps that you should take to maximize your learning while doing. Finally, we'll take an in-depth look at a few of the most common scenarios in which we medical students will be pressed to apply their knowledge.

## Two broad categories of applying

First, some housekeeping. In this section, we distinguish between two categories of activities where you apply your knowledge: **educational activities** and **practical activities**. As medical learners, we are most familiar with educational activities. The aim here is to increase our knowledge or abilities in anticipation of some future real world application in the real world. Examples include practice exam questions, seeing simulated patients, engaging in case-based discussions, attending anatomy lab, and practicing in procedural skills labs (e.g. surgical knot tying). An important subset is academic assessments, such as licensure exams (e.g. USMLE Step 1/2/3 exams) and school-specific requirements.

In contrast, practical activities are those where the major aim is something other than learning, although we do learn as a byproduct. As physicians, our major practical activity is the actual doing of medicine with real patients.

In this section, we will mostly address educational activities, since these activities are likely your major concern at the moment as a medical student. However, the learning system we're setting forth is applicable throughout your career as a physician, and so we will briefly address how to maximize learning from real-life practical activities as well.

Although Apply encompasses a wide variety of different activities, the underlying principles we've discussed throughout this book are well suited for them all.

# Spacing and Interleaving

Application, like studying, benefits from a distributed schedule as opposed to cramming. If you'll recall from *Brain Science*, we discussed studies that looked at the learning of procedural skills in medicine and found that spacing out the practice of those skills enhanced retention and efficiency.[23] Similarly, for cognitive skills, spreading out your application in educational activities (like question banks or cases) will be superior to massing all your application in long bouts.[24]

But apart from the scheduling of practice sessions, the order in which practice activities are performed *within a session* has been shown to matter as well. The idea is called **interleaved practice**. Interleaved practice is "alternating the practice of different kinds of items or problems," as opposed to blocked practice, where items or problems of the same kind are done in succession.[22] For example, let's say you have a practice question set that has 5 questions for each of the following diseases: acute kidney injury (AKI), nephrotic syndrome, glomerulonephritis, and renal cell carcinoma. In total there are 20 questions. If you answered all five AKI questions first, and then did the same for the remaining diseases, this would constitute blocked practice. If, on the other hand, you mixed it up, and did an AKI question, followed by renal cell, and then nephrotic syndrome, and so on, you would be doing interleaved practice.

In the end, you do the same questions, so there shouldn't be a difference in your learning performance, right? Surprisingly, the ordering does matter, and an increasing number of studies point to the conclusion that interleaving is more efficacious than blocking.[22] For example, one seminal study asked college students to compute volumes of different geometric solids (square, cylinder, etc.). One group of students engaged in blocked practice, where all the square questions were attempted first, then the cylinder, and so forth. The other group interleaved these questions, seeing a problem for each kind of solid every four problems. When the college students came back a week later to do two novel problems for each of the solid types, the interleaved group exhibited superior performance, getting ~60% correct vs. ~20% correct in the blocked group.[25]

Recently, the first study of interleaved practice in medicine was conducted, putting this technique in the service of teaching residents to become certified in the fundamentals of laparoscopic surgery (FLS).[26] In this study, the residents were randomly assigned to a blocked practice group or an interleaved group, and each group performed 20 trials for each of four FLS tasks: peg transfer, pattern cut, extracorporeal suture, and intracorporeal suture. Four weeks later, the residents came back to the teaching lab and completed two more trials of each of the four tasks.

On the peg transfer, the interleaved group demonstrated significantly superior performance ($p<0.05$), while for intracorporeal cut tasks and extracorporeal cut tasks, the interleaved group showed a trend ($p>0.05$) toward superior performance, with large effect sizes. Overall, the conclusion of this study is that, in the very real context of laparoscopic surgical training, interleaving practice can have a positive impact.

Implementing this powerful technique is straightforward. For your educational activities, make sure to interleave the kinds of tasks you see. In our example above, we interleaved different disease-related questions *within the same subject*. This kind of within-in-subject interleaving is appropriate for when you're initially learning new material. So, for example, if you had recently acquired new knowledge about renal pathology, and you had a test coming up on renal diseases, then interleaving different kinds of renal questions is the right choice. But, when you have more knowledge under your belt and you are studying for more comprehensive exams such as a shelf, or Step 1 or Step 2CK, then interleaving across subjects would be better. Indeed, many good question banks, give you a random order, where a question pertaining to anything from embryology to biostatistics could pop up at any moment.

Apart from practice questions, you could and should interleave in other educational activities as well. If you were solving clinical cases, you'd want to do diverse case types, rather than all cases of the same type. Similarly, if you were working on building procedural skills, perhaps in your school's simulation center, you'd want to interleave the specific tasks, just as those surgical residents did in the study we discussed above.

In real life, interleaving will happen just as a consequence of the random nature of what kinds of patients present on the wards. If you're rounding with your medicine team, the stop at each patient's room will force you to apply quite different knowledge and skills. The post-stroke patient in one room will prompt you recall knowledge about neuroanatomy and to apply your neuro exam techniques, while the cirrhosis patient in the next room may have you trying to remember the clotting factors and practicing your thoracentesis skills. So in real life, interleaving is built in.

## Practice like the real thing

If you wanted to become a star basketball player, what would be the best use of your time?

(A) Practicing your jump shot
(B) Swimming in the pool at the gym

No doubt, you'd say practicing your jump shot. Swimming might be fun, and maybe it will help your general fitness, but it's not going to make you a great basketball player. The insight here is that if you want to get good at something, your practice should get as close to the real thing as possible.

The same holds true for learning. If we acquire knowledge in order to apply it in particular ways and toward particular ends, then our practice should match those things as closely as possible. Put another way, what we ultimately want to do with our learning is to *transfer* it to a novel yet predictable situation.

One key way to achieve this comes from a concept called Transfer Appropriate Processing (TAP), which states that memory performance will be enhanced to the extent that the processes engaged during initial learning match the processes required for a task.[27] For example, if you wanted to study for a structured exam like Step 1 in a manner consistent with TAP, you'd want to practice with problems that replicate the cognitive processes you'll engage in the real test (gleaning information from clinical vignettes, "two-step thinking," comparing and contrasting multiple choices, etc.) The closer you get the better. Indeed, many students understand this well, which is why there is broad consensus about what the "best" practice resources are: the ones that look like the real test as much as possible.

On the other hand, if you were practicing for a pharmacology class exam that consists of short answer essays where you need to provide justification, you'd do well to replicate that and not spend all your time doing multiple-choice questions. If your aim were to hone a set of procedure skills, say intubating a patient, then TAP would also suggest that you spend more time in the simulation lab practicing intubation rather than just reading about intubation.

Another, related idea, the **Encoding Specificity Principle** states that "memory is improved when information available at encoding, such as external cues, is also available at retrieval.[28] Essentially, this is saying that your context, the environment around you, is an important factor in your ability to retrieve information.

This is one reason why learning new information in clinical environments (clerkships) seems so much better than the classroom. When you're on the wards, you associate new information with the rich environmental cues, as well as your own internal states (e.g. how you feel at the moment, what you were thinking, etc.) Encoding specificity takes most prominence when you're doing practical activities (I.e. actual patient care) than with educational activities, but even with the latter, trying to match your practice environment to the real thing is a good idea.

So, for example, if your goal is to perform at a high level on your school's anatomy practical exam, where you'll be asked to identify anatomy on a cadaver, then the best way to practice applying your knowledge is in the anatomy lab itself. Indeed, savvy med students know this and they come in after hours to practice their anatomy knowledge on cadavers. In this way, they take advantage of all the cues available to them – the sounds, smells, touch, emotions, etc. – that are present in the anatomy lab but not in the library or coffee shop where you study.

# Self-Explanation

Earlier, we introduced the idea of self-explanation as a way to enhance retention and promote understanding. How might you use this technique when you are applying? One prominent place to apply self-explanation is when doing practice problems that have detailed explanations. Most good question banks or workbooks have detailed answers. Rather than just reading those answers, self-explanation would prompt you to account for why each step is taken, what knowledge that step relied on, etc. In the *Preliminaries* section, we provided a list of prompts that are appropriate for just this situation, so refer to that section for guidance.

# Capture new information while applying

When you're working practice questions, or doing a case-based session at school, undoubtedly you're going to pick up new knowledge. These nuggets need to be captured for safe keeping, just like any other piece of information you want to remember. Thus, when you're doing these kinds of educational activities, you should keep some kind of peripheral brain, either your SRS or notes system, to capture new information from application for later review.

From practical activities in the real world, you'll also pick up a lot of new information while you're doing. While you're performing a physical exam in the pediatrics clinic, for example, your preceptor tells you that the red, vascular lesion on your patient's back is a strawberry hemangioma, and that these are fairly common and go away over time. Since you're interested in pediatrics, you capture this pearl on your iPhone and then later put it into Anki. That's acquiring-while-applying and it happens all the time. The key is to have a ubiquitous capture tool, a smartphone or notebook, whatever you'd like, to record this learning. We discuss tools and criteria for capturing information in the Implementation section.

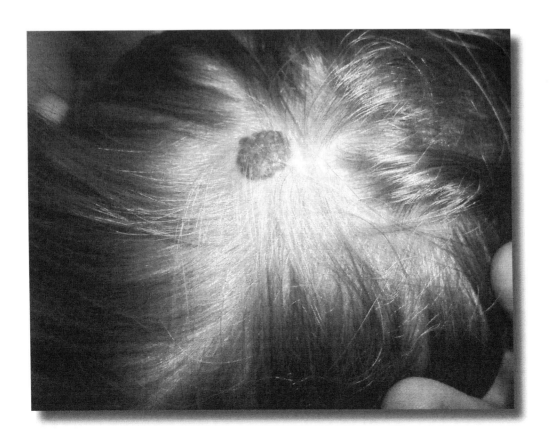

# Be deliberate

There's more to practice than doing the same thing over and over. Psychologist K. Anders Ericsson has written a number of papers around the idea of deliberate practice, and writer Malcolm Gladwell has popularized the "10,000 hour rule" that derives from this line of work. So what is deliberate practice?

Deliberate practice means having a well-defined objective, repeated practice with clear outcome measures, and continuous feedback and monitoring. If you want to get good at something, you have to measure your skill, and keep practicing until that measurement improves. This sort of deliberate practice is goal-directed, and is much more effective at improving performance than rote repetition. Putting in the hours is important, but how you practice matters as much as how much time you spend on it.

Athletes and musicians know this. Basketball stars will practice for hours on making the same shots, over and over, and tracking how many of them they sink. Top musicians, rather than playing through a piece several times, will specifically focus on the trickiest passages and play them until they can get it right on stage. In fact, the best musicians will often sound terrible when they practice, specifically because they keep doing back to the passages where they mess up the most!

How does this apply to medicine? Some elements of deliberate practice are built into our learning system – Anki, for example, gives you instant feedback on whether you've got a question wrong. Deliberate practice can also be a strategy in reviewing practice questions, such as on Step 1. Rather than doing general practice questions, you should keep track of which subjects you are weakest on, and spend time drilling down on those topics. Some programs will automatically break down your performance skills by content area. Don't let this useful information go to waste. Yes, your natural inclination is to spend more time working on the things you know well, since it makes you feel smart and competent. That's good for your ego but not for your performance. Practicing deliberately means focusing on your weak points in a structured and consistent way. The reward for your deflated ego is greater gains in your academic performance.

You can also use deliberate practice to hone your practical skills. Suppose you're learning the physical exam, and you've gotten fairly comfortable with the broad strokes. One common weak point for a lot of students is being able to assess reflexes reliably, especially in the arms. In that case, it would behoove you to buddy up with a classmate (or a very tolerant patient) and practice eliciting the biceps, brachioradialis, and triceps reflex until you're comfortable with it. The same principle applies to the procedural skills you learn in residency; whether it's putting in a central line or performing open-heart surgery, deliberate practice is the best way to become an expert.

More generally, whenever you're practicing a skill, it's important to self-assess after practice to see how you are performing and where you need to improve. Your goal is to watch your performance over time. You want to improve consistently. If you don't see that increasing improvement, then that indicates that something about your strategy needs to change. Getting that feedback is crucial to improving.

# Summary Points: Apply

1. Space out your application over time.
2. Use interleaved practice within study sessions.
3. Match your practice as closely as possible to the actual thing you want to do.
4. Capture new information that you learn while applying into your peripheral brain.
5. Practice deliberately.

# Chapter 13:
## Bringing It Together – An Example Of The Learning Method In Action

We've covered a lot of ground over the last chapters, and you may still be wondering how to implement the practices we've outlined. Thus, to demonstrate the Learning Method in action, we're going to work through a realistic example.

Over the course of three days, our hypothetical med student, let's call her Jessica, is going to cover a large swath of Gastrointestinal (GI) Pathology using the tools of the Learning Method.

Jessica's goals are the same as any medical student's: she needs to pass class, prepare for high stakes board exams, and learn for her future career. At this moment, Jessica has allocated her learning efforts mostly toward Step 1 preparation, since she wants to do well so that she is well positioned to match in any residency. At the same time, her school makes some activities mandatory; so she balances her own independent learning with some class time, which ensures that she can pass her class exams. And, in the process, some of what she learns from Step 1 prep and class will be useful for her career as a physician, but because Jessica doesn't know what she wants to specialize in, she's not fixed on acquiring any particular medical domain knowledge. She just let's her learning for life happen in the background.

Using her broad goals to guide her, Jessica has mapped out a detailed schedule on her calendar for the next three days, from Monday, February 16 to Wednesday, February 18, using our principles to create an actionable study plan. She's divided her independent learning into study blocks of 90 minutes so that she can remain focused and energized while working. She's also made sure to intersperse key breaks in between studying, allocating time for meals, errands and leisure.

Much of Jessica's independent study will take place in the extra room in her apartment that she keeps as an office. This is a quiet place where distractions are limited, allowing her to focus. Here, she has set up a standing workstation so that she can switch between sitting and standing, to help her alertness and promote her health. Jessica does most of her studying on her laptop. To keep her from checking Twitter or Facebook every five minutes, she's using a blocker app such as Self-Control.

Because Jessica has little prior knowledge about GI pathology, she knows that she needs to get the big picture first from high quality, Level 1 introductory source that overlaps well with her learning goals. Then, when she has some background, she can go deeper for more details from more comprehensive sources.

Jessica prefers to learn from videos and text, mixing them for some variety. Using the criteria she learned in *Gather the Right Resources*, she selects Pathoma as her Level 1 resource. With this package, she watches well-made videos with an accompanying text so that she doesn't need to try to furiously capture information for later extraction to her SRS or notes system. After she's completed her Level 1 pass over the material, she'll then move on to a solid Level 2 resource, *Robbins Basic Pathology*, to flesh out the big picture view she got Pathoma. If needed, Jessica will keep a Level 3 resource nearby, such as *Robbins Pathologic Basis of Disease,* but she'll only consult it if something is unclear. Since she doesn't plan on being a pathologist, she decides to leave that information for the specialists.

For each of her study blocks, Jessica has tools to prime her learning. First, she has a framework. In particular, since she's studying Pathology, she'll use her illness framework to help her organize the new information she'll acquire. For some of her learning, especially during Level 2, she'll use the back-of-chapter questions to pre-test herself so as to enhance her uptake of new information.

Jessica has built in dedicated time for initial and maintenance reviews – first thing every morning. This allows just enough time to elapse between learning new information and first reviewing it, consistent with the principle of desirable difficulties. Her maintenance reviews, on the other hand, she does when she has time, but in the evenings before bed. During her reviews, Jessica doesn't just mindlessly answer questions. She thinks about her responses, especially for questions she gets wrong. And she tries to make connections between the knowledge she retrieves so as to promote understanding.

Ultimately, Jessica wants to apply her learning toward specific ends. Accordingly, she builds in application activities that closely match the real setting in which she will apply her knowledge, taking advantage of principles such as transfer appropriate processing, encoding specificity and deliberate practice. Since she is focused primarily on high performance on Step 1, she incorporates several study blocks to do practice questions, such as those from USMLE World. She selectively studies only those questions overlapping with the subject matter she's studying at the moment (GI Pathology), leaving other subjects for a later time.

Jessica wants to be competent when she hits the wards in her clinical clerkships, so she also needs to practice those cognitive and procedural skills she'll use there. Thankfully, her school wisely coordinates a Clinical Skills Course and Simulated Patient session to overlap with the subject matter that she and her classmates are covering in the classroom. Thus, in her clinical skills course, she works on solving cases for common GI pathologies such as appendicitis, inflammatory bowel disease and peptic ulcer disease. In the process, her preceptors guide her in interpreting lab values, radiological evidence and physical exam signs to make her diagnosis. Later in the day, she'll further refine her physical exam and history-taking skills during

## February 2015

| Mon 16 | Tue 17 | Wed 18 |
|---|---|---|
| | | 6 AM Breakfast |
| 7 AM Breakfast | 7 AM Breakfast | 7 AM Do first time review of SR cards from day prior (Feb 17, 2015) |
| 8 AM Do SR Maintenance Reviews | 8 AM Do first time review of SR cards from day prior (Feb 16, 2015) | Drive to School |
| 9 AM Go for a run | | 9 AM Study Block 1: Continue Robbins Basic Pathology Chapter 14 - Or... |
| | Drive to School | |
| 10 AM Study Block 1: Pathoma Videos/ Text 10.1-10.2 | 10 AM Study Block 1: Do (40) USMLE World Qbank questions on GI pathology | 10:30 AM Clinical Skills Course |
| 11:30 AM Lunch | 11:30 AM Pathology Lab | |
| 12:30 PM Small Group Learning at School | | Lunch |
| | 1:30 PM Lunch | 1:30 PM Study Block 2: Pathoma Videos/ Text 10.8 |
| Drive back to A... | 2:30 PM Study Block 2: Robbins Basic Pathology Chapter 14 - Oral Cavity and Gas... | |
| 3 PM Study Block 2: Watch Pathoma Videos/Text 10.3-10.4 | | 3 PM Simulated Patient Session |
| | Drive back to a... | |
| Clean apartment | 4:30 PM Study Block 3: Pathoma Vide... | |
| 5 PM Study Block 3: Watch Pathoma Video/Text 10.5 | | Drive Home |
| | | 5:30 PM Dinner |
| | Dinner | |
| 6:30 PM Dinner | | 6:30 PM Study Block 1: Do (40) USMLE World Qbank questions on GI pathology |
| | 7 PM Do SR Maintenance Reviews | |
| 7:30 PM Finish SR reviews for day | | Chores |
| 8:30 PM Free time | 8:30 PM Watch a movie with friends | 8:30 PM Daily SR Maintenance Review |

a session with a simulated patient presenting with a chief complaint of epigastric pain after eating (cholelithiasis). Taken together, all these activities closely approximate what she'll need to do during her clerkships and beyond.

Let's now take a closer look at a study block from each of the steps of the learning method – Acquire, Review and Apply – to help you see more clearly how all the specific tools come together.

# Acquire

Study Block 2
Monday, February 16, 2015 (3 PM to 4:30 PM)
Material: Pathoma Videos and Text, Section 10.3 (Esophagus) and 10.4 (Stomach)

In this study block, Jessica is going to watch two Pathoma videos and follow along with the accompanying text.

# Priming – (10 minutes)

Before she starts watching the first video, Jessica will prime her mind in several ways. First, she will refer to the text, looking at the section subheadings and turning them into questions to pre-test. If there were end-of-chapter questions, she'd use those, but this particular text doesn't have them, so she's on her own. Jessica turns the subheadings into questions like "What is achalasia?" and "What etiologies can I predict would cause achalasia?" Again, it's okay if she doesn't know all the answers yet – it still primes her to learn the material.

Last but not least, Jessica makes sure she has a framework in mind that can she use to organize the incoming information while she learns. Since she's learning Pathology, she uses the Disease Framework (see *Implementation*), which contains mental 'slots' for items like time course, etiology, pathogenesis, sign and symptoms, etc.

# Watching – (50 minutes)

Now that's she ready to acquire, Jessica begins to watch video 10.3 on the esophagus. She has the accompanying text open while she watches the video so that she can make any annotations of information that is said in the video but not written in the text. Since most of the annotation is already done for her (by the text), she can watch the video at 1.5x speed, helping her move more quickly.

Since each video contains within it multiple diseases, Jessica pauses the video after each disease. She does this for a few reasons. One is that she wants to check her understanding, stopping to define new terms or clarifying confusing ideas before moving on. The other reason is that she knows that she can combat lapses in her attention by interspersing some active learning, for example, by posing questions to herself about what she just learned (e.g. "What are the clinical features of GERD"). She also uses the self-explanation prompts that she learned in earlier sections of this book. In total, she aims to spend about 30-60s pausing and reflecting before moving on.

After video 10.3 is over, she goes back to the text to add any additional information she gleaned from the video, and she identifies facts that will go into her SRS. Since this is a Level 1 resource tailored to Step 1, most if not all the information will be high-yield for Jessica's purposes. Therefore, she refrains from highlighting the whole book, but rather she knows that she'll go back at the end of her study block and extract many facts into her SRS. Jessica then repeats the same process for video 10.4.

## Extract to SRS – (~20 minutes)

Jessica captures the facts from the Pathoma text into Anki, using the guidelines she picked up in the 'How to Make Cards' section. She'll review these cards when she does her initial review the next morning. For now, she's just getting the information into her SRS.

It's worth noting here that card making takes time 20 minutes of Jessica's time. Although there is value in selecting the particular information that goes into your SRS there is also a time cost. If Jessica could use cards that were already made for her that overlap well with her resources, it would be a huge efficiency gain for her to use these, since she could learn knowing that SRS cards would be waiting for her at the end. It's worth inquiring with upperclassmen or checking the commercial SRS options to see what options for premade cards are available.

## Reflect – (10 minutes)

In the remaining time in her study block, Jessica wants to organize her thoughts and make connections between the things she's learned. Referring to tools she learned in the

*Think and Organize* section of this book, she decides to make a simple flow diagram of the knowledge she acquired from her studying. Importantly, she focuses on making relationships and categorizations that are not directly from the book, but that she notices herself. For example, several of the esophageal diseases she learned were due to aberrant anatomy, and so she grouped them as together. Moreover, she realized that some of the non-malignant esophageal diseases could be risk factors for eventual malignancies, so she represented those connections. Jessica doesn't try to capture everything she learned on this diagram. She records the highlights, trying first to produce a graph from memory, and then checking its accuracy against her book. In this way, she gets the benefit of retrieval practice in addition to the enhancement she gets from organizing her thoughts.

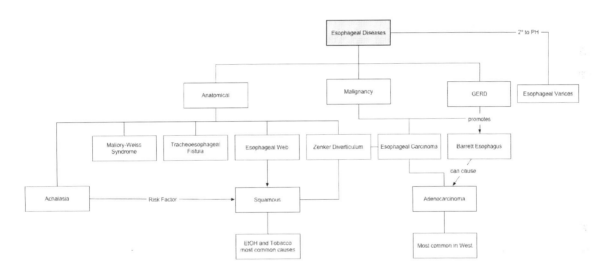

When she makes her Level 2 pass at this same subject matter, she can return to fill in additional details she learns.

# Review

## Initial review

Tuesday, February 17, 2015 (7:00 to 8:00 am)

After learning a lot of new material the previous day (Monday the 16th), Jessica knows that she must now do her initial review to halt the rapid forgetting that will likely happen otherwise. She's placed this initial review on the next morning and not immediately after her studying, since she wants to take advantage of the idea of desirable difficulties.

To begin, she fires up Anki on her mobile device and takes her work outside, walking around her quiet neighborhood while she does her reviews.

Here is a sample from Jessica's initial review.

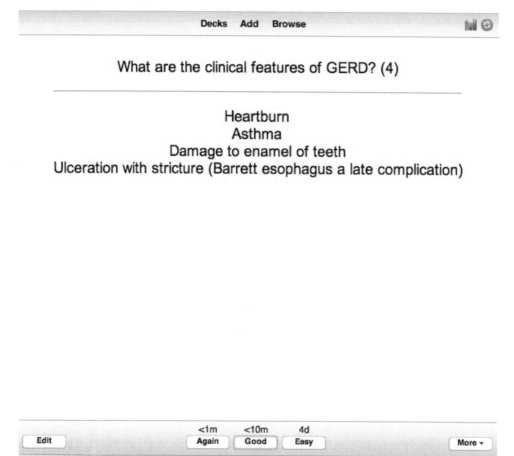

Because she's cognizant of the way that review loads can pile up, she limits herself to a maximum of 100 new facts in this initial review. This means that not all of the newly minted SRS cards she made the day prior (Mon 16th) will be reviewed at this time. Rather, Jessica will put off the remainder of her new Level 1 SRS cards for a later time, most likely tomorrow morning. She does this because she knows that her Level 2 learning from Tuesday will not produce nearly as many new SRS cards as her Level 1 learning.

"But won't Jessica forget the things she learned on yesterday if she doesn't review them today?" Most likely, yes, but that's the trade-off she has to make since she doesn't want to do 200 or 300 new SRS cards in one day and then get swamped with those reviews at a later time in her maintenance reviews. The saving grace is that in her Level 2 learning today, she will re-study much of the material she learned on yesterday's Level 1 resources. This will refresh her memory of the things she learned the day prior, helping her to effectively 'reset' her forgetting curve.

Although this sounds complicated, Jessica doesn't really have to think about it. She sets her daily new card limit in Anki to 100, and then just let the app do the rest.

During her review, Jessica makes sure to think about the answers she gives, and when she answer incorrectly, she takes time to think about her answer in relation to the correct one, noting the differences.

At the end, she takes a few moments to reflect further on the whole of the knowledge she retrieved. In particular, she tries to connect her learnings, comparing and contrasting the different disease entities, which will ultimately enhance her ability to engage in efficient diagnostic reasoning in the clinic.

# Maintenance review

Tuesday February 17, 2015 (7:00 to 8:30 pm)

In addition to reviewing new information in her initial review, Jessica also has to maintain to retain. So, every day, she must perform a maintenance review, which consists of all the SRS cards she's learned in the past, presented at the appropriately timed interval based on her prior performance.

There is nothing complicated about this review. It just needs to get done. So, Jessica gets comfortable on the couch in her apartment and fires up Anki, navigates to her Pa-

+ Pathology Deck          172          150

thology deck and sees the number of reviews due today (172). And then she does them, thoughtfully and with focus.

# Apply

Wednesday February 18, 2015 (6:30 to 8:00 PM)
Study Block 3: Do (40) USMLE World Qbank Questions on GI Pathology

With new knowledge in mind, Jessica is now ready to begin to apply her learning. Because she's gearing up for Step 1, she's using material that closely matches the real thing, choosing a well-regarded question bank from USMLE World. Just as in the other steps, before she starts doing practice questions, she makes sure she's got a game plan and is in a setting where she can focus.

To focus on practice questions that overlap with her recent learning, she uses the features of the qbank to selectively study GI pathology. After Jessica answers each question, she takes time to read the detailed explanation. If she answered the question correctly and with ease, she moves more quickly through the explanation, just to see if her reasoning was accurate. When she gets questions wrong, she moves more slowly through the detailed explanations. She applies the self-explanation prompts she learned for worked examples, which guides her through understanding the correct answer and helps her to update her knowledge. Lastly, if the explanation reveals gaps in her knowledge – facts or ideas she didn't know – she captures that information into her SRS or notes system so she can retain that knowledge. This is an example of acquiring-while-applying or learning by doing.

Jessica also makes sure to flag or mark the questions she gets wrong, since these are the kinds of questions she'll need to focus on if she wants to practice deliberately. Good tools like USMLEWorld allow students like Jessica to track their progress and analyze where their efforts should be directed. At a later point, perhaps before her upcoming class exam, Jessica will use this knowledge to focus selectively on concepts and questions that she consistently gets wrong. This kind of deliberate and focused practice on weak points is the potent ingredient that helps people build expertise. Moreover, by using analytic tools to monitor performance, Jessica can see how her performance changes over time, helping her to refine and redirect her efforts in way that is consistent with her goals.

# Learn, Practice, Repeat

So that's how you put the Learning Method into practice. We offer this example as a template for your own implementation, but we definitely recommend that you tweak the methods to best fit your needs.

In the end, the Learning Method could be summarized in this one liner: "Learn, practice, repeat." If you ever find yourself getting lost in the weeds of all the tools we've given you, just remember this mantra. At the core is the simple idea that you need to get things into your head, and then keep them there through review (spaced retrieval practice) and application. Learn, practice, repeat.

# References For Section III – Learning Method

1. Anders Ericsson, K. Deliberate Practice and Acquisition of Expert Performance: A General Overview. *Academic Emergency Medicine* **15,** 988–994 (2008).

2. Moulaert, V., Verwijnen, M. G. M., Rikers, R. & Scherpbier, A. J. J. A. The effects of deliberate practice in undergraduate medical education – Moulaert – 2004 – Medical Education – Wiley Online Library. *Medical Education* **38,** 1044–1052 (2004).

3. Green, M., Jones, P. & Thomas, J. X., Jr. Selection Criteria for Residency: Results of a National Program Directors Survey. *Academic Medicine* **84,** 362–367 (2009).

4. Bunce, D. M., Flens, E. A. & Neiles, K. Y. How Long Can Students Pay Attention in Class? A Study of Student Attention Decline Using Clickers. *Journal of Chemical Education* (2010). doi:10.1021/ed100409p

5. Lavie, P. Ultradian rhythms in alertness – a pupillometric study. *Biol Psychol* **9,** 49–62 (1979).

6. LaJambe, C. M. & Brown, F. M. in *Ultradian Rhythms from Molecules to Mind* 283–301 (Springer Netherlands, 2008). doi:10.1007/978-1-4020-8352-5_13

7. Ericsson, K. A., Krampe, R. T. & Tesch-Römer, C. The role of deliberate practice in the acquisition of expert performance. *Psychological Review* 100, 363–406 (1993).

8. Patel, A. V. *et al.* Leisure time spent sitting in relation to total mortality in a prospective cohort of US adults. *American Journal of Epidemiology* 172, 419–429 (2010).

9. MacEwen, B. T., MacDonald, D. J. & Burr, J. F. A systematic review of standing and treadmill desks in the workplace. – PubMed – NCBI. *Preventive Medicine* 70, 50–58 (2015).

10. Dutta, N., Koepp, G., Stovitz, S., Levine, J. & Pereira, M. Using Sit-Stand Worksta- tions to Decrease Sedentary Time in Office Workers: A Randomized Crossover Trial. *International Journal of Environmental Research and Public Health 2014, Vol. 11, Pages 9361-9375* 11, 6653–6665 (2014).

11. Labonté-LeMoyne, É. *et al.* The delayed effect of treadmill desk usage on recall and attention. *Computers in Human Behavior* 46, 1–5 (2015).

12. Monsell, S. Task switching. *Trends Cogn. Sci. (Regul. Ed.)* 7, 134–140 (2003).

13. Mayer, R. E. Applying the science of learning to medical education. *Medical Educa- tion* 44, 543–549 (2010).

14. Dunlosky, J., Rawson, K. A., Marsh, E. J., Nathan, M. J. & Willingham, D. T. Im- proving Students' Learning With Effective Learning Techniques. *psi.sagepub.com*

15. Larsen, D. P., Butler, A. C. & Roediger, H. L. Comparative effects of test-enhanced learning and self-explanation on long-term retention. *Medical Education* 47, 674– 682 (2013).

16. Chi, M. T., De Leeuw, N., Chiu, M.-H. & LaVancher, C. Eliciting self-explanations improves understanding. *Cogn Sci* 18, 439–477 (1994).

17. Hausmann, R. G., Nokes, T. J., VanLehn, K. & Gershman, S. The design of self-ex- planation prompts: The fit hypothesis. 2626–2631 (2009).

18. Conati, C. & VanLehn, K. Toward Computer-Based Support of Meta-Cognitive Skills: a Computational Framework to Coach Self-Explanation. *International Journal of Artificial Intelligence in Education (IJAIED)* 11, 389–415 (2000).

19. Nokes, T. J., Hausmann, R. & VanLehn, K. Testing the instructional fit hypothesis: the case of self-explanation prompts – Springer. *Instr Sci* (2011).

20. Larsen, D. P., Butler, A. C., Lawson, A. L. & Roediger, H. L. The importance of seeing the patient: test-enhanced learning with standardized patients and written tests improves clinical application of knowledge. *Adv in Health Sci Educ* (2012). doi:10.1007/s10459-012-9379-7

21. Bjork, R. A. Memory and metamemory considerations in the training of human beings. (1994).

22. Dunn, D. S., Saville, B. K. & Baker, S. C. Evidence-based teaching: Tools and tech- niques that promote learning in the psychology classroom. *Australian Journal of Psychology* 65, 5–13 (2013).

23. Spruit, E. N., Band, G. P. H. & Hamming, J. F. Increasing efficiency of surgical training: effects of spacing practice on skill acquisition and retention in laparoscopy training. *Surg Endosc* (2014). doi:10.1007/s00464-014-3931-x

24. Carpenter, S. K., Cepeda, N. J., Rohrer, D., Kang, S. H. K. & Pashler, H. Using spacing to enhance diverse forms of learning: Review of recent research and implications for instruction. *Educational Psychology Review* 1–10 (2012). doi:10.1007/s10648-012-9205-z

25. Rohrer, D. & Taylor, K. The shuffling of mathematics problems improves learning. *Instr Sci* (2007). doi:10.1007/s11251-007-9015-8

26. Goldin, S. B. *et al.* FLS skill acquisition: a comparison of blocked vs interleaved practice. *Journal of Surgical Education* 71, 506–512 (2014).

27. Butler, A. C. Repeated testing produces superior transfer of learning relative to repeated studying. *Journal of Experimental Psychology: Learning, Memory, and Cognition* 36, 1118–1133 (2010).

28. Lieberman, D. A. *Human Learning and Memory*. (Cambridge University Press, 2012).

29. Carey, B. (2014). Why Flunking Exams Is Actually a Good Thing. *New York Times*.

30. Grimaldi, P.J., and Karpicke, J.D. (2012). When and why do retrieval attempts enhance subsequent encoding? *Mem Cogn* 40, 505–513.

31. Brown, P.C., Roediger, H.L., and McDaniel, M.A. (2014). *Make It Stick* (Harvard University Press).

# Section IV
## Implementation

# Chapter 14:
## Implementation – An Overview

Up until now, we've been talking about general principles and tools for learning. But without guidance, it's hard to turn that theory into practice. So in this section, we're going to take these building blocks and turn them into actionable study plans for medical school.

We're going to break down each medical school discipline and give you a study strategy tailored for that subject. We'll bring some perspective to this study plan by analyzing which parts of each subject are most important for boards and clinical practice, and deciding which areas you should pay extra attention to and which can be safely crammed and forgotten.

We'll also recommend major resources (beyond the ever-valuable *First Aid*) that we and our classmates found most useful when we were learning these subjects. Many of these resources we recommend are already popular, others are more obscure but equally valuable. Finally, we'll present sample study schedules for each subject, so that you can keep up a sustainable pace – and approach subjects in the right order – if you choose to study on your own.

We hope you find these resources helpful, but keep in mind that every medical school is different. We based our study schedule on Duke's curriculum, which has a fair number of idiosyncrasies, such as doing all our preclinical courses in first year. Likewise, the resources we present are those that we and our classmates were most familiar with. So take these specific recommendations as a guideline. If some of them are not a great fit for your school's unique circumstances, tailor them accordingly.

# The importance of frameworks

Medicine has its own internal logic, but our course materials don't always reflect that elegance. In most medical schools, unlike in college, a single course will have multiple lecturers, who don't always coordinate together. In the worst cases, what we learn from lectures lacks any overarching principles, and devolves to just memorizing a random assortment of facts. Textbooks tend to be better, since they're written in advance, but even they are not always organized in the best way to help you learn what you need. So it's ultimately each student's job to make sure he has a good conceptual framework to learn each subject. That's where we come in.

In the following chapters, we'll devote considerable space to sketching out frameworks to help you make sense of each of these topics. For example, we'll show you how to think about classes of drugs together, as a unit, so that the logic of each drug class becomes clear and you not just memorizing lists of meaningless syllables. Having the right frameworks will help you follow the internal logic of each subject, making your learning more engaging and more efficient. The more we structure our learning to reflect the way this knowledge is used on exams and in clinical practice, the better we'll be at recalling and applying our knowledge in the real world.

# Our first recommendation: Skipping class responsibly!

There are three main ways to acquire information in med school. You can attend lecture in person, stream online, or study on your own, referring to the curriculum only for general guidance.

Each of these options has merit. Which one(s) you choose depends on your goals and your circumstances. If you want to ace your school exams, then using lecture slides, video and class notes as your primary sources would be the best option, since they're made by the same people who are writing your exams. On the other hand, if you're prime concern is board exam preparation, studying high-yield review books would be superior, since they are focused on preparing you for the board exam. Your personal preferences matter, too. Some people can't stand textbooks, but they enjoy hearing someone teach live or on video.

Med school is different from college – the pace of learning is more intense, and the way classes are set up is often very different. And so, you may find that the tried-and-true ways that you learned in college have to be adapted for med school.

That's why we recommend taking the few weeks at the beginning of first year, before things really ramp up, as an opportunity to experiment and find the way of learning the best suits you. Schools know that everyone is still adjusting to medical school, and they almost always make the first block pass-fail, or at least severely downweight the importance of grades in the first few weeks.

So go to class in person for a few days, then try streaming lectures at home. Finish up by trying to follow along with textbooks or review books. You're going to be spending a lot of time learning in medical school, and figuring out the right habits at the beginning of the year will pay dividends for the rest of your med school career. This time, before med school gets too intense, is your chance to experiment, make mistakes, and find the learning methods that will serve you well the rest of your med school career. So make use of it.

> "Figuring out the right habits at the beginning of the year will pay dividends for the rest of your med school career."

# Chapter 15:
# Anatomy

Anatomy is the quintessential med student class, the class that brings out the skeleton in front of the classroom, and puts you through the rite of passage that is the cadaver lab. It's also a clinically important subject, as the intricate construction of the human body forms the basis of many specialties, from surgery to radiology.

At the same time, it's one of the most challenging subjects in medical school. It brings in a huge body of information that most students haven't even started learning in undergrad. Furthermore, a lot of the information is about 3D relationships that can only imperfectly be captured on the pages of Gray's Anatomy. So a systematic approach can be very helpful here.

## Framework

Anatomy is a visual discipline, and is best approached by breaking the body down into regions. Instead of first learning the entire musculoskeletal system, then the GI tract, and so on, we should break the body down into thorax, abdomen, arm, leg, and so on. All the organ systems affect one another; the nerves innervate the musculoskeletal system, the blood vessels supply the organs, and so on. By learning the body *regionally* you can see how structures from different organ systems interrelate. Fortunately, most schools do take this approach.

Another challenge in learning anatomy is that when we get down to the level of individual muscles, nerves, and vessels, the volume of information can be overwhelming.

Every organ is connected to a web of nerves and vessels; every muscle passes over some structures and under others. That's why it's important to have a good framework so that when you see a structure, you can instantly recognize the relevant facts.

To cut through the noise, you should recognize that every type of structure has a particular set of facts associated with it. For example, for every blood vessel, you'll want to know what vessel it arises from, what its branches are, and what region it supplies blood to. Now that you know that, every time you see a blood vessel in a textbook, you can zoom in on that information. This will help focus your learning and make the information overload less overwhelming.

To extend this concept, whenever you see a **muscle**, you should think about the following information:

- Origin
- Insertion
- Innervation
- Blood Supply
- Function


Every **nerve** should have the following information:

- Origin
- Branches
- Innervation region
- Type of innervation (sensory, motor, or both)


Every **bone** should have the following information:

- Connection to other bones
- Muscle insertion points


Again, every **blood vessel** should have the following information:

- Source
- Branches
- Organs and muscles supplied

And finally, every **organ** should have the following information:

- Blood supply
- Innervation (if applicable)
- Function

# Anatomy tables

This framework may not capture all of the information about human anatomy – most notably, it leaves out information about the spatial relationships between different structures; which vessels pass over which muscles, and so on. But it does capture the vast majority of testable information in a very predictable form. And with this framework, you can go into any part of the body and create tables capturing this information. Here's what a sample muscle table might look like, as demonstrated by a website from the University of Michigan:

**Muscles of the Upper Limb - Listed Alphabetically**

| Muscle | Origin | Insertion | Action | Innervation | Artery | Notes | Image |
|---|---|---|---|---|---|---|---|
| abductor digiti minimi (hand) | pisiform | base of the proximal phalanx of the 5th digit on its ulnar side | abducts the 5th digit | deep branch of the ulnar nerve | ulnar a. | abductor digiti minimi, flexor digiti minimi brevis, and opponens digiti minimi are located in the hypothenar compartment of the hand | |
| abductor pollicis brevis | flexor retinaculum, scaphoid, trapezium | base of the proximal phalanx of the first digit | abducts thumb | recurrent branch of median nerve | superficial palmar br. of the radial a. | abductor pollicis brevis, flexor pollicis brevis, and opponens pollicis are located in the thenar compartment of the hand (Latin: pollicis = the thumb) | |
| abductor pollicis longus | middle one-third of the posterior surface of the radius, interosseous membrane, mid-portion of posterolateral ulna | radial side of the base of the first metacarpal | abducts the thumb at carpometacarpal joint | radial nerve, deep branch | posterior interosseous a. | the tendons of abductor pollicis longus and extensor pollicis brevis make the lateral border of the anatomical snuffbox (Latin: pollicis = the thumb) | |
| adductor pollicis | oblique head: capitate and base of the 2nd and 3rd metacarpals; transverse head: shaft of the 3rd metacarpal | base of the proximal phalanx of the thumb | adducts the thumb | ulnar nerve, deep branch | deep palmar arterial arch | deep palmar arch and deep ulnar nerve pass between the two heads of adductor pollicis, which is in the adductor-interosseous compartment (Latin: pollicis = the thumb) | |
| anconeus | lateral epicondyle of the humerus | lateral side of the olecranon and the upper one-fourth of the ulna | extends the forearm | nerve to anconeus, from the radial nerve | interosseous recurrent a. | (Greek: anconeus = elbow) | |
| biceps brachii | short head: tip of the coracoid process of the scapula; long head: supraglenoid tubercle of the scapula | tuberosity of the radius | flexes the forearm, flexes arm (long head), supinates | musculocutaneous nerve (C5,6) | brachial a. | a powerful supinator only if the elbow is flexed | |
| brachialis | anterior surface of the lower one-half of the humerus and the associated intermuscular septa | coronoid process of the ulna | flexes the forearm | musculocutaneous nerve (C5,6) | brachial a., radial recurrent a. | a powerful flexor | |
| brachioradialis | upper two-thirds of the lateral | lateral side of the base of the | flexes the elbow, assists in pronation & | radial nerve | radial recurrent | although brachioradialis is | |

Figure: Sample muscle table. Source: http://www.med.umich.edu/lrc/coursepages/m1/anatomy2010/html/anatomytables/muscles_alpha.html

Compact, efficient, and to the point, these tables make great reference sheets for later review. They're also a great foundation on which to make flashcards. In the above example, you might make cards asking what the origin, insertion, action, and innervation of each of these hand muscles are.

# Image occlusion

Anatomy is also a good opportunity to introduce a technique that will serve you well in other subjects: image occlusion.

In this technique, you take figures that convey important visual information, and blank out the captions. Your job is to identify structures based on the figure. For subjects like anatomy and biochemistry, this can be an efficient way to learn. To create such a card, first find a labeled figure you like (you can often find relevant figures online). This becomes the "answer" side of the card. To create the question, simply copy the image into Microsoft Paint (Windows) or Paintbrush (Mac) and black out the caption you want to quiz yourself on. Remember to turn on "Fill" option so that the box will obscure the caption. Here is an example of a figure we might want to learn, and the occluded version of the the same figure.

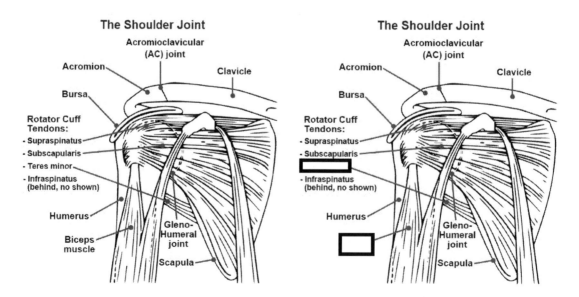

Remember the **principle to quiz yourself on one fact per card**. This applies to image occlusion as well. Don't create a card where you blank out all the captions, and then quiz yourself on all the captions at once. You'll have too many facts on a single card and won't be able to separate out what you know and don't know. In the interests of reducing the burden of making cards, we may relax this rule just a little bit, and let you can bump it up to two or three. In our example above, we blanked out just two of the many structures.

# Resources

## Acland's Videos

This is a video series by a professor of surgery in Louisville who created very detailed expert dissections of cadavers for anatomy. This video series is available by subscription; several medical schools have purchased subscriptions for their students, or you may have to purchase it yourself. Regardless, it's an excellent tool for the visual learner. You get a 3D understanding of structures that is more realistic than the false-color structures you'll find in books, yet clearer and cleaner than what you'll be able to produce in anatomy lab.

## Gray's Anatomy (and Other Atlases)

No, we're talking about the textbook, not the TV show! There are several similar textbooks of human anatomy, and Gray's and Netter's are two of the most popular. They go into great detail about the anatomy, broken down by region of the body. They are very useful as a reference but go into too much detail to be a good resource for primary learning. Like Acland's videos, the best way to use these atlases is to have them open to the region of the body that you're learning, and refer to the detailed illustrations to get a good visual sense of how all the structures fit together.

## The Big Picture: Gross Anatomy

This textbook strikes a good balance between conciseness and thoroughness, and is our recommended resource for primary learning in anatomy. Organized by organ system, it gives a level of detail appropriate for medical school, hitting all of the important testable points without getting bogged down in the nitty-gritty. When we've needed a quick refresher on anatomy later on in med school, such as before a case in surgery, we've referred back to The Big Picture.

## First Aid for USMLE Step 1 ("First Aid")

*First Aid* doesn't have a dedicated section for anatomy, but does address anatomy as a subsection in its organ system chapters. These sections are brief highlights of important, testable concepts; one might cover the cranial nerves, while another covers the arterial supply of the digestive tract. This organization makes it not the best choice for primary learning or even orienting yourself around anatomy. However, you should review these sections after learning the relevant part of anatomy, and be sure to make cards of the high-yield factoids in *First Aid*.

# How do you use anatomy lab?

First of all, don't panic. Dissecting a cadaver sounds scary, and it might be at first, but generations of medical students have gone through it before without a problem. After the initial shock, most people quickly get used to dissecting. In our experience, the speed with which anatomy lab started seeming normal was more remarkable than the fact that we were dissecting a cadaver!

Let's think about anatomy lab's purpose. The most helpful thing anatomy lab can do for you is give you visual and kinesthetic reinforcement of what you've been learning. It's useful to learn anatomy from a book, but physically and visually examining the relationships between anatomic structures in real life can help to reinforce that memory through multiple sensory modalities.

On the other hand, it doesn't work well to do your primary learning off a cadaver. Structures aren't neatly labeled, and you might get confused as to whether something is a nerve or a blood vessel. (Vessels aren't colored blue and red in real life!) You might also have a cadaver with a variant of normal anatomy.

So the way to get the most out of anatomy lab is to go in already having learned the region you're about to dissect. Watch the Acland's videos or read the relevant chapter of your textbook before you go into lab, and use the lab itself as a super-high impact review of what you've learned.

> "The way to get the most out of anatomy lab is to go in already having learned the region you're about to dissect."

Oh, and don't worry too much about messing up structures or achieving a perfect dissection. The intent of anatomy lab is to give you a chance to learn by observing and appreciating the structures that you've been learning about by books; it's not to turn you into a perfect anatomist or perfecting your scalpel skills. As long as you're able to get good review learning from the lab, it has served its purpose.

# Methodology

Your schedule for learning anatomy will likely be determined by your school's anatomy lab schedule. One common way the schedule could be set up is to have a lecture on an anatomic region in the morning or the day before, and the corresponding anatomy lab in the afternoon. We recommend, however, that you start learning the relevant anatomy the day *before* the relevant anatomy lab, so that you can have a sense of what you're doing in lab, and treat the session as a visual review.

So, the day before, sit down with *Big Picture Gross Anatomy* and go over that region of the body. Have *Gray's* on hand as a reference if you get confused, but focus on learning the material in The Big Picture, using the "anatomy table" framework. Another useful technique is to try to reproduce important figures from memory. So, for example, to study the arterial supply of the GI tract, you might draw out the stomach and intestines and mark out what region is supplied by which arteries. This helps you take advantage of the testing effect and reinforces your learning more strongly than if you were merely skimming the page.

Once you're done, flip to the relevant section of *First Aid* and make additional Anki cards out of all the facts listed there. Add in anything else you feel is important from The Big Picture. With this knowledge in hand, you're ready to go into anatomy lab, using the opportunity to experience and test yourself on what you just learned through dissecting the cadaver.

# Sample study schedule

## Week 1
This is a light week, with only one relatively simple anatomic region (the back) to learn. Take the opportunity to get oriented, get all your learning materials together, and get used to thinking anatomically. Topics:
- Back muscles
- Vertebrae
- Spinal cord, roots, and nerves

## Week 2
Thorax, part 1
- Anterior thorax wall muscles and skeleton
- Breast
- Diaphragm
- Lung

## Week 3
Thorax, part 2
- Heart
- Mediastinum
- Thoracic arteries and veins

## Week 4
Abdomen, part 1
- Abdominal wall
- Esophagus, stomach, pancreas, liver, spleen, peritoneum

## Week 5
Abdomen, part 2
- Small and large intestine
- Kidneys
- Innervation and vascular supply of abdomen

## Week 6

Pelvis

- Muscles of pelvis
- Perineum
- Male and female reproductive system

## Week 7

Head, part 1

- Skull, scalp, meninges
- Brain
- Cranial nerves

## Week 8

Head, part 2

- Bones and muscles of face
- Eye, ear
- Nose
- Oral cavity

## Week 9

Neck

- Muscles of neck
- Pharynx
- Larynx
- Thyroid and parathyroid

## Week 10

Upper limb

- Shoulder
- Arm, forearm, hand (muscles, nerves, vessels)
- Brachial plexus

## Week 11

Lower limb

- Hip
- Thigh, leg, foot (muscles, nerves, vessels)

## Week 12

Review, prepare for final exam

# Chapter 16: Biochemistry

Biochemistry is, for better or worse, one of the lower yield topics you'll find in med school. There will be a lot that you're asked to memorize, but only a limited amount of that has clinical relevance. Although there are some logical linkages between the various pathways you will learn, biochemistry is overall heavier on memorization and lighter on conceptual understanding. But the topic does get a fair amount of face time on Step 1, so it's worth learning thoroughly for exam time despite its eccentricities. Fortunately, there are ways to leverage Anki and other learning techniques to maximize your retention of the important facts of biochemistry.

## Framework

The core unit of biochemistry is the biochemical pathway. Whether it's the citric acid cycle, heme synthesis pathway, or the sorbitol formation and degradation pathway, each pathway is a discrete unit of facts that make sense as a unit. There is the basic sequence of reactions and the enzymes that catalyze them. There is the set of regulatory factors that up- or down-regulate the pathway. There is the pathology – the way that a malfunction of this pathway can cause disease. And there may also be pharmacology – the way that drugs might regulate this pathway. There's a lot to learn, but it all starts to make sense when you really understand the pathway.

To understand a pathway, it's helpful to think *teleologically* – to think about what the pathway's purpose is in keeping the body functioning. Let's take the cholesterol pathway as an example.

## What does it do?

It takes up cholesterol, both that found in the diet and that synthesized in the liver. It packages it into VLDL, which drops off cholesterol and fatty acids in the tissues. Eventually the VLDL turns into LDL, which is absorbed by peripheral cells. At the same time, the liver also produces HDL, which takes up any unneeded cholesterol in the tissues and brings it back to the liver.

So overall, the goal of this process is to take cholesterol from the diet and deliver it into the body where it's needed, and take back cholesterol when it's not needed. This broad understanding of the pathway's overall "goal" can guide our learning of the biochemical steps involved.

## What happens when its regulation becomes deranged?

If the liver is unable to create VLDL particles, then instead of being funneled into LDL particles, cholesterol will be stuck in particles that are precursors to VLDL (called chylomicrons). This, as it turns out, is the mechanism of certain familial lipodystrophies – inherited diseases of cholesterol metabolism. At the same time, if the liver creates too many VLDL particles, you'll end up with too much cholesterol going out to body tissues, which can cause atherosclerosis. So you'd expect VLDL creation to be tightly linked with cholesterol inflows from the diet and from liver synthesis, as well as to the cholesterol needs of the body.

## When might you want to have a drug affecting this pathway? What would the effects be?

Cholesterol is a major driver of coronary artery disease and stroke, so there are many drugs that target this pathway. The statin drugs, for instance, inhibit the liver's internal production of cholesterol. Niacin, a vitamin that can also be used as a drug, reduces the production of VLDL. Ezetimibe is a drug that blocks the absorption of cholesterol in the intestine.

Now that we've worked through the cholesterol pathway, it makes intuitive sense that these drugs have the effect that they do on cholesterol deposition in the arteries. This linkage makes it easier for you to remember the biochemistry of the pathways, and understanding the drug mechanisms will give you a leg up when it comes time to learn pharmacology.

It does take a bit longer to get this intuitive understanding, rather than just memorizing a flowchart. But breaking information down by pathways will ultimately help you learn the cluster of facts around each pathway faster, and this will set up you up for long-term sustainable memory.

## What not to learn

Biochemistry has so many molecules and strange names that a lot of it can be overwhelming. As we mentioned, the important thing to understand about each pathway is its teleology: that is, the main points and what it's trying to accomplish. A lot of these pathways will have components that are unrelated to any of these two things. For example, in the glycolysis pathway, there are several steps between fructose-1,6-bisphosphate and pyruvate which are not important regulatory steps, and which are pretty much interchangeable. Memorizing these molecules is low yield. Your exams may go into some detail on these molecules, but if that is the case, these are facts that can be safely crammed and forgotten. The important thing to commit to your long-term memory is what glycolysis is, the products, and the key regulatory steps.

# Resources

## Lippincott's Biochemistry

This is a good text for primary learning, and a reference for when you have detailed questions. It generally goes into more detail than you need for the boards, but for a subject like biochemistry, that additional detail is actually valuable for making sure you understand the teleology and function of each pathway as you learn it.

## First Aid

*First Aid* has a dense but concise chapter on biochemistry. As usual for *First Aid*, it's not enough to learn from, but is a good resource to understand which facts are most likely to be on Step 1. It also has some good diagrams of major biochemical pathways which can be good material for image occlusion flashcards.

# Methodology

As we discussed above, we recommend a pathway-centric approach as you delve into biochemistry. When a pathway is covered in class, before trying to memorize anything, open up Lippencott to the relevant chapter and try to understand the logic of the pathway. Think about its function, its regulation, and its potential role in disease and pharmacology.

Only when you understand all this should you start making cards. As always, *First Aid* is a good guide to what's card-worthy. When you do want to memorize important regulatory steps in a pathway, image occlusion, which we covered in the previous chapter, can be a powerful way to learn biochemical pathways.

# Sample study schedule

### Week 1

Review energy metabolism, which you should have learn a little about in college biochem. Topics:
- Glycolysis
- Gluconeogenesis
- TCA cycle
- Krebs cycle
- Electron transport
- Relevant metabolic disorders

### Week 2

The rest of metabolism, using *First Aid* as a guide. Topics:
- Glycogen processing
- Urea cycle
- Fructose, galactose processing
- Relevant diseases

### Week 3

Finishing up metabolism
- Lipids, ketones, cholesterol
- Secondary pathways (Cori cycle, HMP shunt, sorbitol)

### Week 4

Molecular biology and genetics. Topics:
- Inheritance patterns
- Common genetic diseases (and their inheritance patterns)
- DNA/RNA production and salvage
- Protein synthesis
- Molecular biology techniques

## Week 5

Cellular biochemistry, nutrition
- Cellular biochemistry: mitosis, cellular structures, related diseases
- Vitamins: functions, deficiency diseases, toxicity diseases

## Week 6

Miscellaneous metabolism
- Catecholamine synthesis
- Amino acid derivatives
- Various diseases (e.g. phenylketonuria)

# Chapter 17: Physiology

Physiology is the study of the mechanical and chemical interactions that allow the body to operate normally. Simply put, it's the story of how the body *works*. It encompasses the hormone systems of the body, as well as diverse topics such as kidney filtration and maintaining blood pH. (Finally, your chemistry prereqs will come in handy!)

Learning physiology can be challenging because of its breadth, but many of our classmates found it to be their favorite subject because many of these mechanisms make elegant sense. The surface details may appear complicated, but as you learn them, you'll come to realize the deeper logic of why the body works the way it does. More than most subjects, physiology rewards conceptual understanding over rote memorization, and our study strategies reflect that.

## Framework

As with biochemistry, the unit of analysis here is a single system, such as the thyroid hormone system or the self-regulation of the cardiac cycle. And, as in biochemistry, teleologic thinking can be a valuable framework to use in learning physiologic pathways. You can think of each system as having a particular goal, and having the regulatory systems and feedback that help it to achieve that goal. For example, the thyroid hormone system seeks to have a tightly controlled, appropriate amount of thyroid hormone floating around, and will have feedback based on sensing whether the body's drifting towards a hyper- or hypo-thyroid state. Unlike biochemistry, though, the systems of physiology are simpler, involving less abstruse memorization. Almost every step in a physiologic pathway actually makes sense as part of what makes the system function.

Once you absorb the logic behind each system, it will become easier to think through the logic of the *diseases* that disturb those systems. To continue our example, there are a variety of diseases, such as Grave's disease or Hashimoto thyroiditis, that increase or decrease the body's production of thyroid hormone. If you don't have a framework, you'll have to learn about each of their individual mechanisms and physiologic effects separately. If you do have a framework, however, you can easily figure out their effects by simple logic. For example, Grave's disease is an autoimmune disease causing oversecretion of thyroid hormone, so its symptoms are the obvious things you'd expect with too much thyroid hormone, such as diarrhea, heat intolerance, weight loss, and hair loss. Without the understanding how the thyroid hormone system works, you'd have to memorize an apparently random bunch of facts; with the physiologic understanding, everything falls in place.

We're usually pretty agnostic about learning from books versus lectures, but physiology is one case where we firmly come down on the side of books. Because physiology puts a premium on deep understanding, it's worth a lot to be learning from well-organized books, where you can sit down and learn a pathway in one go.

# Resources

## BRS Physiology or Physiology (Costanzo)

BRS Physiology is the reigning king of review books for physiology. Despite being called a board review book, it goes into significantly more detail than most, and it's thorough enough to use for primary learning. While it does go into more detail than you need for the board exams, it does it with a thoroughness that will ensure your understanding of the material. In a subject like physiology, this will pay dividends down the line. And so, we recommend that you use this book as the source of primary learning for physiology.

If you want more detail, an excellent Level 2 version of BRS Physiology is Physiology by the same author, Linda Costanzo. Many of our classmates have raved about this book, benefiting from the extra depth it offers.

## First Aid

*First Aid* covers some basic physiology in its chapters. It's a good source of material to make cards from, but is not adequate for primary learning, particularly since learning physiology focuses more on understanding than on memorization. Use *First Aid* only as a review source, to make sure you haven't missed anything. If you have any questions, refer back to BRS Physiology.

# Methodology

As we've emphasized, physiology is best approached system by system, and rewards deep understanding over memorization. For this reason, we recommend that you follow read BRS Physiology methodically, section by section. You can either follow the book's organization, or read the appropriate sections as they're covered in lectures. Either way, don't move on from a section until you understand the purpose, regulation, and components of the system you're studying.

Once you're sure you understand one system, refer to *First Aid* and make cards for the relevant facts. Just like in anatomy and biochemistry, image occlusion is an easy way to create cards that test your knowledge of the steps in various pathways. Cards that test your knowledge of regulatory mechanisms are also important.

You may notice that we're recommending more thorough learning here in physiology than we do in most other topics. We're encouraging you to learn more deeply, deeper than is strictly needed for board exams. The reason is that in this particular subject, extra effort goes a long way, for two reasons. Not only does understanding physiology pay off in terms of long-term retention, it also provides a solid grounding that will help you learn pathology and other subjects later on in med school.

# Sample study schedule

**Week 1**

Cellular physiology and respiratory physiology

- Osmosis
- Acid/base balance

**Week 2**

Neuromuscular physiology

- Action potentials
- Neuromuscular transmission
- Muscle contraction (skeletal, smooth, cardiac)
- Temperature regulation

**Week 3**

Cardiovascular

- Review of cardiac electrophysiology and muscle function
- Cardiac cycle
- Blood pressure regulation
- Shock

**Week 4**

Respiratory

- Gas exchange and transport
- Ventilation and perfusion
- Respiratory control

**Week 5**

Renal

- Renal electrolyte handling
- Regulatory hormones
- Acid-base balance
- Diuretics (a nice preview for pharmacology)

**Week 6**

Endocrine

- Pituitary hormones
- Thyroid
- Adrenals
- Insulin and glucagon
- Calcium regulation
- Male and female reproductive hormones

# Chapter 18:
## Pharmacology

There's a game called "Drug or Pokemon?" that works exactly as you'd expect. After showing you a word, it'll ask you whether it sounds more like an antiarrythmic drug or a cute cartoon character with a silly name. And as it turns out, it's actually a pretty tough game.

And that sums up why pharmacology can be so challenging. You're essentially given a list of arbitrary drug names, with no particular hook or framework to aid memory, and asked to memorize some facts about those drugs. And in med school, as with Pokemon, you gotta catch 'em all.

Fortunately, we have the tools to deal with that. Anki can help us remember even strings of random syllables – recall that it was originally developed to learn vocabulary for a foreign language. And there's a right way to organize all this information to bring pharmacology together logically. With this framework, we can achieve deeper understanding even as we make the task of memorizing that list of names easier.

## Framework

In pharmacology, you've got to learn the names, mechanisms, clinical uses, and side effects of over a hundred drugs. This information is laid out clearly, drug by drug, in any pharmacology textbook. So, at least the challenge in front of us is clear. Even with Anki, it would be incredibly painful to just learn this massive table of facts. Much smarter is trying to find organizing principles here that are not arbitrary, that actually make sense.

For pharmacology, this means focusing on mechanisms, and all the drugs using any particular mechanism as a single unit first. That way, you can focus your effort on remembering the *general* traits of each drug class, and then learn the small individual variations that make drugs of this class unique. Even better, once you understand the mechanism, often the side effects make logical sense, which further reduces your burden of memorization.

Let's use beta blockers as an example. *First Aid* will tell you that you have a bunch of drugs in that category. You've got **acebutolol**, **betaxolol**, **esmolol**, **atenolol**, **metoprolol**, **propranolol**, **timolol**, **pindolol**, and **labetalol**. (The book also helpfully points out that they all end in -lol.)

That's actually fantastic, because instead of learning each of these nine drugs individually, you can learn about their effects *as a class*, since they all work by a similar mechanism. So you can then learn that any of these nine drugs can be used for hypertension, myocardial infarction, and superventricular tachycardia. And you can then go on to break them down into still smaller mechanistic groupings, such as the two drugs that happen to be nonselective alpha- and beta-agonists: carvedilol and labetalol. And once you understand how the beta receptors work (among other things, they increase the heart rate and dilating the bronchi), it makes total sense that beta blockers would cause bradycardia (slow heart rate) worsen any asthma symptoms a patient might have. Now, instead of having nine random names, each with a bunch of random facts attached, we have a single drug class whose actions make logical sense.

So that's the way to break down pharmacology into manageable chunks. You'll be learning hundreds of drugs, but they really only fall into a few dozen categories. Once you learn the categories, you've got a really solid foundation in pharmacology, and you can then fine-tune your knowledge by learning the little quirks of individual drugs.

*First Aid* and Katzung both helpfully break down their pharmacology sections into mechanistic categories. Use them.

# Resources

## Katzung and Trevor's Pharmacology: Examination and Board Review

This is a thorough textbook that covers all major drugs and drug classes in exhaustive fashion. Drugs are organized by mechanism and each is described by its mechanisms, effects, clinical uses, and side effects. This is a fine book for primary learning. It gives enough detail to make the underlying logic of each drug class clear, and has tables to organize all this information. However, it goes into too much detail to be used directly as a source of flashcards.

## First Aid

*First Aid*, on the other hand, gives just the bare bones. In its pharmacology chapter, as well as in subsections in all the organ system chapters, it lists out all of the drugs that are likely to show up on Step 1. For each drug, it gives a few words on mechanism, clinical use, and side effects. Because it is so terse, it leaves out a lot of information about mechanisms that can help to tie together your learning. Thus, it's not a great resource for primary learning. But it's useful both as a review and as a reference during your first pass on Katzung and Trevor to inform you of which facts are boards-worthy.

# Methodology

Although lectures may be useful to lay out a framework for understanding broad drug classes, the bulk of the work in pharmacology is straightforward memorization which is best done from books.

Before you even begin, it's helpful to learn the rules for drug suffixes. Often, all drugs of the same class have the same suffix by convention. For example, all beta blockers end in –lol, so every time you see a –lol suffix, you automatically know what kind of drug that is. Knowing these rules can help reduce the load of memorization going for-

> "The bulk of the work in pharmacology is straightforward memorization which is best done from books."

ward. So before you start seriously diving into pharmacology, it's a good idea to look in the *First Aid* pharmacology chapter, find the table laying out these suffix rules, and convert it into Anki cards.

Now, to work. Our preferred methodology is to break drugs down into categories by mechanism. So, you might study all the antidepressants at once, or learn all the anticoagulation drugs in one sitting, depending on what's being covered in class.

Once you've picked your category, start reading Katzung and Trevor to understand both the normal physiology that the drugs act upon, and the broad outlines of how these drugs work. For example, how does coagulation work, and what are different mechanisms by which drugs might be able to prevent coagulation? Then, with a framework in mind, carefully read about the drugs in this class, keeping in mind similarities and differences. Finally, once you're comfortable with your understanding of these drugs, fire up Anki and make cards from *First Aid*.

One important thing to keep in mind is not to learn too many drugs at once. Pharmacology is very dense, and learning more than a dozen drugs at one sitting is asking for trouble. "Antidepressants" or "antipsychotic drugs" is a reasonable category of drugs to learn in one sitting, but "all psychiatric drugs" – which covers over fifty drugs with diverse mechanisms – is asking too much. You can start getting all the drug names mixed up, or worse yet, fail to understand the difference between different drug categories. Pace yourself, learn a moderate amount every day, and keep up with your reviews – that's the way to attack this mountain of information.

A final note: pharmacology is a great topic for collaborative card-making efforts. The kind of cards you make are very mechanical, and so it's easy for a group of classmates to divide up the work of making cards and produce a deck that can be used by everyone. We managed to organize such a group at Duke and this helped us save considerable time in our studying.

# Sample study schedule

## Week 1

Drug suffices and autonomic drugs. An ambitious start, since there are a lot of drugs that fall into these six categories, but this exercise will reinforce the value of learning drugs in terms of categories rather than as individual drugs

- Learn the drug suffixes
- Cholinergics and anticholinergics
- Alpha agonists, beta agonists
- Alpha blockers, beta blockers

## Week 2

Cardiovascular drugs

- Calcium channel blockers
- Other vasodilators
- Diuretics
- ACE inhibitors and aldosterone blockers

## Week 3

Respiratory drugs

- Antihistimines
- Prostaglandins
- Bronchodilators
- Serotonin agonists and antagonists

## Week 4

CNS drugs, part 1

- Barbiturates and benzodiazepines
- Antiseizure drugs
- General and local anesthetics
- Opioids

## Week 5

CNS drugs, part 2

- Antiparkinson drugs
- Antipsychotics
- Antidepressants

## Week 6

Hematologic drugs

- Anticoagulants
- Growth factors
- NSAIDs and immunosuppressants

## Week 7

Endocrine drugs, part 1

- Pituitary hormone drugs
- Thyroid and antithyroid drugs
- Corticosteroids
- Gonadal hormones

## Week 8

Endocrine drugs, part 2

- Insulin and other antidiabetic drugs
- Bisphosphonates
- Lipid drugs

## Week 9

Antibiotics, part 1

- Antibacterials (there are a lot of different classes of antibiotics!)

## Week 10

Antibiotics, part 2

- Antimycobacterial drugs
- Antifungals
- Antivirals

## Week 11

Miscellaneous drugs
- Antiparasitics
- Chelators and antidotes
- Chemotherapy drugs

## Week 12

Review

# Chapter 19: Pathology

If physiology is the study of how the body regulates itself normally, pathology is its dark reflection – the study of how the body can malfunction in disease. Pathology is one of the most useful subjects you'll study in the preclinical years. Many of the topics you'll study here are diseases that you'll see on the wards and in your future practice, and are foundational no matter what specialty you go into. It's also a high-yield section to study for Step 1, because it serves as a point to integrate knowledge from other topics, from biochemistry to pharmacology. In fact, it's so high yield that many Step 1 review courses, such as Goljan's audio lectures and Pathoma, focus entirely on pathology. Rather than covering all the medical school subjects separately, they zoom in on pathology and use it to tie together key points from all the other preclinical subjects.

## Framework

In textbooks, pathology is organized into organ systems, and within each organ system it's broken down into several different pathologic processes. It's tempting to accept this framework and study pathology as a list of diseases that can afflict different organ systems.

In practice, this isn't the best idea. In real life, and on board exams, you're not only asked to rattle off a string of unconnected facts about disease, but rather to *differentiate* between distinct diseases that present similarly. For example, you might get a case about a patient who presents with shortness of breath, then be asked whether this the disease in question is asthma or heart failure. In that case, what you'd want to be able to do is recognize that asthma and heart failure are two diseases that can cause shortness of breath, and then know how to differentiate between the two. Merely knowing the list of symptoms of asthma and heart failure is not as useful. Most often, on tests and in clinical practice, you're playing compare and contrast. Your studying should reflect that.

"Most often, on tests and in clinical practice, you're playing compare and contrast."

That's where the **disease framework** comes in. Whenever you learn about a new disease, also start thinking about the cluster of facts that helps you differentiate it from any other, similar diseases. This cluster might include important symptoms, important "negatives" (for instance, a heart attack usually does not present with wheezing, and absence of wheezing can help differentiate a heart attack from asthma.) It can also include lab values and radiologic tests. By thinking in terms of this framework, you'll develop pattern recognition for each illness's particular "script," which you can then compare and contrast with other diseases. The ultimate goal is that when you hear about a case, whether on Step 1 or on the wards, you'll be able to mentally run through a list of potential diseases, figure out the key differentiating factors that will help you decide between them, and zero in on the most likely disease.

There is no single way to incorporate the illness framework into your learning. The most important thing is to approach your learning with this orientation in mind, keeping an eye to playing "compare and contrast" whenever you hear about diseases with similar symptoms. One simple strategy is to create flashcards whenever you think of important ways to distinguish between two similar diseases. For instance, you might make a card "What physical exam findings distinguish asthma from myocardial infarction?" "Asthma has expiratory wheezes." Or perhaps "What lab finding distinguishes asthma from myocardial infarction?" "MI has elevated cardiac enzymes." With these cards, rather than memorizing long list of symptoms and laboratory findings, you're zeroing in on the important things you'll need to know when you have to decide when a patient has one disease or another.

Another approach that some students have used is to create a master spreadsheet containing the vital information for each disease that they learn about. The columns could include things like "symptoms," "lab tests," "physical exam findings," and so on. This gets all of your data in one place, which is both convenient for later review and allows you to make comparisons between different diseases at a glance. The other feature of the spreadsheet approach is that it's extendable. In your pathology course you can start filling it out by including disease presentations and pathophysiology. Later in your med school career, when you start thinking about treatment and therapies, you can add additional columns to complete your knowledge about each disease. This emphasizes the continuity of your medical studies.

# Resources

## Pathoma

This is a newer video and textbook course that has become an overnight cult classic. It contains both a lecture series and an accompanying textbook by a pathologist from the University of Chicago. It strikes a good balance in terms of detail and conciseness, and many students have found it a valuable resource for both board review and primary learning of pathology.

## First Aid

*First Aid* has a thorough set of entries for pathology, split between a dedicated pathology chapter and subsections within individual organ system chapters. As with other subjects, it's not complete enough to do primary learning from, but is a fine source for Anki-worthy material.

## Robbins Basic Pathology

Also known as "Baby Robbins," this classic textbook is written at a good level for medical school learning, and is a good resource for primary learning of pathology. It has detailed explanations and figures for almost all the material that is likely to come up in medical school.

## Step Up To Medicine

This is a review book for the wards and Step 2 CK exam, but can be useful in learning pathology as well. What it adds to the picture is an understanding of how the material you're learning can be applied clinically. We recommend this as an optional supplement when reading one of the other textbooks. This book will also come in handy later in your career when you're studying for Step 2.

# Robbins and Cotran's Pathologic Basis of Disease

This is a full-length pathology textbook, the full version of "Baby Robbins" above. It's a classic, often used even by pathology residents, and is broad and inclusive. But it goes into too much detail to be used as a primary learning resource. However, it can serve as a good reference.

# Harrison's Principles of Internal Medicine

This is the classic internal medicine counterpart to Robbins, a staple of medicine residents. Like "Big Robbins," it's too dense to study from, but can be used for a more clinically-oriented review. Most hospital libraries will have a copy, so if you intend to refer to it once in a while, there's no need to purchase this monster and lug it around.

# Methodology

For all its complexity, the process of learning pathology is relatively straightforward. Open Baby Robbins or Pathoma to the section that you want to learn. Have *First Aid* open to the corresponding section. Read through the subsection in Baby Robbins, highlighting as you go. (If you're using Pathoma, watch the relevant video subsection, taking notes as you go.) When you finish the subsection, use the highlighted portions (or your notes) to create Anki cards and to fill in information on your illness spreadsheet. Then proceed to the next section until you're done with your learning session. At the end of your learning session, go to *First Aid* and capture any factoids not gleaned from your reading.

For review questions, we recommend Robbins Review of Pathology. It is an excellent source of practice questions that will really test your knowledge of pathology. Moreover, it maps seamlessly with Robbins Basic Pathology, with specific page references and all. As medical students we used this book to very good effect, as did our classmates. The problems are significantly harder than those you'll see on the USMLE Step 1, so if you can answer these questions, you'll be poised for success on the pathology questions on Step 1. It is even likely that your professors will use this book to guide their exam question design. Other worthwhile tools include USMLE World questions for Step 1.

Many schools also have adopted small group problem solving sessions for pathology. These can be very valuable; not only is it a chance to review, but it's a format that mimics the way you'll see cases in real life. They're good opportunities to test out your skills and practice thinking like a clinician.

# Sample study schedule

This is a fairly compressed schedule, 20 weeks long, reflecting our curriculum at Duke. This pace is doable, but takes significant discipline and efficiency, which is why we developed the efficient learning system we've described above. At many schools, pathology is spread over an entire year. If that's the case for you, you can space out your studying accordingly, and take more time to dive into the details.

**Week 1**
- General inflammation and repair
- Hemodynamics, shock

**Week 2**
- Coagulation disorders

**Week 3**
- Immune disorders
- General principles of cancer

**Week 4**
- Genetic diseases
- Environmental diseases
- Nutritional deficiencies

**Week 5**
- Cardiovascular disease, part 1

**Week 6**
- Cardiovascular disease, part 2

**Week 7**
- Pulmonary disease, part 1

**Week 8**
- Pulmonary disease, part 2

**Week 9**
- Renal disease, part 1

**Week 10**
- Renal disease, part 2

**Week 11**
- Hematopoeitic diseases

**Week 12**
- Gastrointestinal disease, part 1

**Week 13**
- Gastrointestinal disease, part 2

## Week 14
- Hepatic and pancreatic disease

## Week 15
- Male and female reproductive diseases

## Week 16
- Breast disease
- Lower urinary tract disease

## Week 17
- Endocrine diseases
- Musculoskeletal diseases

## Week 18
- Central nervous system disease

## Week 19
- Peripheral nervous system disease

## Week 20
- Skin diseases
- Review

# Chapter 20:
## Clinical Skills

Depending on the school you go to, you may or may not get a great deal of teaching on clinical skills before you hit the wards. These important clinical skills include interviewing patients to get the story of what's been going on, performing a physical exam, and "soft skills" involving motivating patients and communicating effectively with patients and other physicians.

Some schools go into great detail on these skills; others merely give a brief overview of the physical exam. Some of you may be in clinical skills classes that treat the topic briefly, or that don't teach it well. Although they'll play a role in Step 2 CS, none of these skills will show up on Step 1.

Nevertheless, these skills are going to prove essential to your ability to do your job as a physician, long after your ability to recite the citric acid cycle is nothing more than a parlor trick. So it's worth spending a little extra effort now, above and beyond what your school may require, to practice and perfect these skills. After all, eliciting signs and symptoms is a major part of what the job of "doctoring" is all about!

## Framework

Many of these skills fall under procedural memories – they're about knowing how to do things rather than just recalling facts. As such, flashcards have some limited utility, but most of your "studying" here will involve practice. But while Anki may not pay a central role, it's still important to bear in mind the principles we introduced in *Brain Science*.

The most important thing to do to perfect and retain these skills is to practice whenever you can. Counsel patients, interview them, and do physical exams, whenever you have an opportunity. If you don't have regular patient contact as part of your course, practice the physical exam on yourself and on your friends until it becomes second nature. You can think of this as sort of spaced repetition that you're running on yourself, training the essential procedural memories required for these clinical skills. And because you're practicing these skills in real-world environments, you're taking advantage of transfer-appropriate processing, so that the skills will transfer to when you're taking care of patients independently.

Anki comes in handy when you're first learning physical exam techniques. Useful cards include those that ask you about the steps of the physical exam in a particular region. Special physical exam techniques – like Kernig's sign that is a classic test for bacterial meningitis – merit their own cards. The goal here is to build up memories of what tests are appropriate in which situations.

# Resources

## Bates' Guide to the Physical Examination and History-Taking

This is a pocket-sized book that gives a good grounding for physical exam and interview skills. It gives step-by-step descriptions of each exam step and maneuver, sorted by organ system and with helpful images. You can use it as a pocket reference on the wards, or work through it slowly as a simple textbook hitting the major points.

## YouTube videos

The physical exam is, well, physical, and that's something that can be hard to convey through text or even figures. Fortunately, there are a large number of high-quality videos online for every physical exam maneuver. Videos are a good resource if you need to review a particular maneuver, or figure out how to perform it on a patient. For example, if you have a patient with a knee injury, and remember from your reading that you want to perform an anterior drawer test to test for ligament damage, you can look up how to perform that test, then go into the room and do it.

## JAMA's Rational Clinical Exam

This unique online resource, which your school likely subscribes to, is arranged differently than most textbooks. It's set up by clinical question, not by organ systems. If you have a particular patient presentation, it can tell you the high-yield physical exam steps that will help you come to a firm diagnosis. One unique feature is that it is evidence-based; it gives quantitative assessments of how likely diseases are given particular presentations, and how helpful different exam findings are to pinpoint your diagnosis. So it won't give you unhelpful tips or obsolete historical curiosities, but rather just what you need to get the clinical answers you want.

# Methodology

Again, the key to learning the physical exam is practice. Therefore, it makes most sense to concentrate your studying when you'll have a chance to practice on patients. Many schools have a dedicated physical exam block where you'll get a chance to study the physical exam. This is the first time it makes sense to dedicate time to studying the physical exam. During this time, use Bates as a reference to guide your studying. Make flashcards of specific maneuvers and tests, so that you have them in your head when needed.

But most importantly, use muscle memory to remember the sequence of actions for each region of the clinical exam. Perform each step over and over until it becomes second nature. For example, for the abdominal exam, you might observe, auscultate, palpate, percuss, palpate the liver edge, palpate the spleen, and palpate the aorta. At first doing all this will feel like checking items off a checklist, and you'll have to think through each step. As you practice this over and over, though, it will become automatic, and by the time you're seeing patients on your own you won't have to think about it. Furthermore, performing the actions will cement it much better than reading this list off an Anki card

During your clinical year, make a conscious effort to practice a thorough physical exam. That year is also a good time to deepen your knowledge of the physical exam beyond what was taught in your formal course. You can carry Bates in your pocket and use it along with Youtube videos as references to make your exam more though and precise. For example, instead of merely listening for the heartbeat for any murmurs, you can learn the different areas of the chest where different valve sounds are the loudest, and identify the different types of heart murmurs. Attendings and residents will often ask you what you want to learn; asking for a demonstration of particular physical exam techniques or time to practice these is always a good idea. Finally, when patients present with complaints, you can use the Rational Clinical Exam site to map out the most important exam steps to perform in that particular patient. In time, your exam will become more precise and be mindful rather than robotic.

# Chapter 21:
## USMLE Step 1

Time to put your game face on. Step 1 is *the* high-stakes test of medical school, the biggest test of your preclinical knowledge. It is one of the top criteria, if not *the* top criterion, for most residency applications. For better or worse, for many of you, it will be the goal you've been striving towards for two years of medical school.

The good news is that all your hard work during your preclinical years pays off in this crucial moment. Most students, using conventional study techniques, will come into this study period having forgotten a great deal of what they learned earlier. They'll need to spend a large fraction of their Step 1 study time just re-learning this knowledge. On the other hand, your hard work learning and retaining knowledge with Anki means that you have a solid stock of knowledge in your head even before you sit down to study specifically for Step 1. You don't have to cram a ton of content; you can focus almost all of your time on practice questions, directly getting better at taking the test.

There are many books and resources that specialize in helping you tackle this beast, and we'll discuss some of them below. Our goal here, though, is not to delve deep into the nitty-gritty, but to present an overall strategy that can guide both your immediate study period as well as your two years of preclinical learning.

Our recommendations are going to look a little different from most of the study plans out there, because your solid preclinical preparation opens up more freedom in how you approach your study. As we mentioned, you have the unique advantage of not needing to do in depth content review. You'll be able to use this freed-up time to do additional question review, which will greatly improve your score. So don't worry if what we recommend looks different from what you see some other students doing. You're simply starting from an advantageous position, and with our plan, you'll do even better!

# Know your foe

The USMLE Step 1 is eight hours long (including one hour of break time) and contains about 322 multiple-choice questions. Anything from the preclinical years is fair game. You won't be asked to give a detailed treatment protocol of *M. pneumoniae* (they save that for Step 2 and 3), but you'll certainly be asked anything they can think of about its biochemistry, microbiology, immunology, or pharmacology.

Framed this way, your goal should clearly be to have as much preclinical knowledge in your head on test day as possible. That's why we've recommended that you use *First Aid* – a book with a concise summary of everything likely to be on the test – as the backbone of your preclinical studying.

It's also time to revisit our "no cramming" attitude. Recall back in the *Brain Science* section that we typically shunned cramming because it buys you better short-term retention at the expense of long-term retention. But here, with a high-stakes test looming, our goal is to have as much in our memory the day of the test, regardless of what happens after. So there is a role for some cramming in this process.

# Resources

## USMLE World

"UWorld," as it's affectionately known, is far and away the best question bank out there. It contains over 2,000 high-yield questions written in the same style as real board exam questions. Even better, each question comes with a detailed explanation of why one answer is right and the others are wrong. Because of its fidelity to the actual exam, as well as the detailed explanations that are great for studying and flashcard making, we recommend that you make this question bank for the backbone of your studying. You should certainly aim to complete this question bank during your study period, and review the questions that you got wrong.

## NBME Practice Tests

These are official tests from the National Board of Medical Examiners based largely on retired questions that have been on previous iterations of Step 1. They can be useful to get an idea of what the test is like – each is about half the length of a full Step 1 exam and gives you a three-digit score analogous to a Step 1 score. However, unlike in UWorld, there is no explanation of which questions you got wrong, only a list of your strengths and weaknesses in different subject areas. For an extra $10 NBME will identify the questions you got wrong, but will not indicate the correct answer or explain the reasoning that led to that decision. If you're looking for a predictor of your score, these tests are the best place to get it. However, because of its lack of explanations, taking this test won't help you gain a stronger foundation in the actual test topics. Therefore, we suggest that you use these tests only as a diagnostic, if you must use them at all.

## First Aid and Textbooks

As always, you will have *First Aid* and your other textbooks available for references, but beyond a quick browse through *First Aid*, we don't recommend spending a lot of time doing primary studying using these resources. Much of this knowledge should already be in your head, so using the question banks should be a much better use of time.

## Other Question Banks

Kaplan and other companies have come out with question banks as well. Although these are similar in form to UWorld, we found them to be less helpful. Some of them are too detailed for the real test, and many of them lack key features such as detailed analysis of the questions that you got wrong. As a result, we generally recommend that you stick with in-depth UWorld reviews rather than roam further for additional question banks.

# How to study

Depending on your school, you'll get between 4 and 8 weeks of dedicated time to study for this exam. Here's a list of action items to make the most of your time. There may be other tools you'd like to use, and you can insert them into this plan appropriately. We've tried to keep our recommendations to the simplest, most effective strategies.

Before you do anything else, sit down and plan out your study period. Figure out how much time you have, and plan out how much time you want to dedicate to each of the phases we'll outline below. This is important to avoid misallocating your study time, or worse yet, running out of time before test day.

Here is one plan for how you might use your time, assuming six weeks to study. In the rest of this section, we'll explain each of these steps, which should form the backbone of your study plan. Given your time constraints and self-assessment of your performance, you may wish to adjust the order of activities and the proportion of time spent on each. This is fine, as long as you end up actually completing each of these important activities.

# Sample study schedule

Throughout: Continue reviewing Anki cards

**Week 1:** NBME practice exam, *First Aid* review

**Week 2:** *First Aid* review

**Week 3:** USMLE World review, adding flashcards to cram deck

**Week 4:** USMLE World review, adding flashcards to cram deck

**Week 5:** USMLE World review, adding flashcards to cram deck

**Week 6:** USMLE World review, review cram deck

**3 days before test day:** Memorize "cram and forget" material

**2 days before test day:** Memorize "cram and forget" material

**1 day before test day:** Light Anki review and rest

## 1. Continue reviewing Anki cards

Remember that Anki shows you facts as you are about to forget them. While all the other review strategies in this list are important and high yield, none of them will be as attuned to your individual memory curve as your personal flashcard deck. So keeping up with Anki remains a high-yield activity.

## 2. NBME practice exam

In our plan, we recommend taking one NBME practice exam. The purpose here is to have a very rough estimate of how prepared you are before you start studying. If you score well here, it can give you peace of mind and reassure you that your need for content review is fairly minimal. If you score poorly, you may benefit from some more focused content review as well as doing review questions.

However, don't overestimate the predictive value of the NBME exam. These exams vary quite a bit in difficulty, and many people score significantly better or worse than their NBME results suggested. These scores are best viewed as *rough* estimates of your knowledge base, with error bars of perhaps +/- 15 points or so. Furthermore, although your score report will claim to show relative strengths and weaknesses by subject area, in reality there are so few questions within each subject area that this information is not very useful to help focus your studying. In statistical terms, the test is too "underpowered" to detect any actual variation in your understanding of different areas.

For that reason, we recommend only a single NBME exam at the beginning of your studying, and only for rough calibration purposes. Some people take multiple exams over the course of their study period to try to gauge their progress, but we don't recommend this. We have much better uses of your time lined up…

## 3. Review weak spots

We recommend doing a high-level walk through of *First Aid*, looking for weak spots and stopping to learn from review books when you've found a topic you're shaky on. If you've been making and reviewing cards for all preclinical subjects, this shouldn't take too long, since most of this stuff should be in your memory. But nobody is perfect, and now's a great chance to review old weaknesses.

One good way to do this review is to cover up all the text except for the subject headings, and try to recreate all the content from memory. So you might open up to the heading "Hydralazine" and remind yourself of all the facts you know about hydralazine. Then uncover the text and see what additional facts you may not have remembered. This is a fast way to incorporate the testing effect into your review.

Most importantly, pace yourself. Make sure this review is high level, and make it fast – a week or two is a good goal. We want to preserve the bulk of our study time for practice questions, which brings us to our next item.

## 4. Complete the UWorld question bank

UWorld is a great resource, not only for getting you familiar with the format of the test, but also to ingrain the important topics and angles that the USMLE likes to emphasize. Step 1 is idiosyncratic. It has a few specific facts that it likes to emphasize over and over. For example, in anatomy, it loves to quiz you on the fact that palsy of the long thoracic nerve can cause winged scapula. This question bank can help focus your studying towards the most important topics. For this reason, completing it is our top priority, and we dedicated the majority of your test prep time to doing so.

UWorld can be sorted by subject area, so it may be worthwhile to combine your UWorld review with your *First Aid* overview to hit topics at the same time, if you so choose. It can also be done in a timed mode that simulates the pace you'll have to keep on the test. This important feature can help you learn the rhythm of the test, to ensure you won't run out of time on test day.

You can also recruit the power of Anki to enhance your UWorld study. Before you start your reviews, create a new deck called "UWorld." Whenever you get a question wrong, create a card in this deck. After you're done with UWorld, review the deck in cram mode, rather than in spaced repetition mode. The purpose of this deck isn't to maintain memory for the long haul, as with your preclinical cards. Rather, you'll use it as a handy base of facts that you can cram quickly right before the exam. Writing the facts in Anki form also gives you a learning boost from exploiting the testing effect, as compared to if you merely kept notes on a cram sheet somewhere.

One final note. Some students found it useful to review UWorld questions during the preclinical years as an additional form of practice. If you did this, make sure to put enough time (a few months) between when you first reviewed them for class and when you're reviewing them for boards. That way, your reviews will be testing your clinical knowledge, rather than memory of irrelevant facts ("Oh, I remember that question about the 46-year-old woman was about cholecystitis!")

## 5. Cram the remainder

For better or worse, everyone has some weak areas that must be crammed. In fact, it's best to figure out early on in your studies which subjects or subsections need to be thoroughly learned and which can be safely crammed. The ideal subjects to cram are those that do not interrelate with other. Some examples include biochemical pathways, embryological sequences, obscure groups of parasites, and niche drugs. Such subjects are best addressed by the "memorize and forget" strategy. Mark these areas or keep a note sheet so that when cramming time comes, you can learn all these facts in one sitting.

Remember the principles from the *Brain Science* chapter. Forgetting happens quickly after the first review. So it's important to cram as close to test day as possible. And active review – asking questions of yourself, and the like – is still the superior study strategy for cramming.

# For test day

This eight-hour exam is definitely a marathon, not a sprint. You have seven hours of solid test time, plus one hour of break. Here's some tips to help get you through it.

## 1. Reconnoiter

If time permits, check out the location beforehand. Make sure you can find it on test day; check out the traffic on the way there. Some test centers will even let you do a trial run, for a fee. They'll let you take the tutorial on their computers, as well as verify your ID information and show you the locker area. This is probably excessive, but it's an option.

## 2. Take the tutorial

NBME offers an online version of the computer tutorial that's shown on exam day. It's worth going to the NBME website and reviewing this tutorial during your study period. This will get you acclimated to the test environment without contributing to fatigue or eyestrain on test day itself. As a bonus, you'll then be able to skip the tutorial on test day, and that will net you a valuable 15 minutes of extra break time.

## 3. Pack snacks

You'll be there all day, and there's no lunch break. So pack some energy dense food so you can chow down fast and keep yourself going. Some energy bars or nuts would work well here. Also pack a few bottles of water to keep yourself hydrated.

## 4. Take breaks

The test offers you one break after each testing block. Some people are tempted to skip these breaks to plow through the test and get it over with sooner. That's usually a bad idea. Taking the test isn't fun, but you've spent two years studying for this, and it's silly to take shortcuts now that might cost you a few points. Take at least a short break at each opportunity. Walk around, take some deep breaths, and let your brain recharge.

## 5. Celebrate!

No matter how you feel. You've just finished what's perhaps *the* biggest exam of your life, and passed a major milestone on your path to becoming a doctor. Go celebrate and relax a while before med school revs up again.

# Chapter 22:
## On The Wards

There's good news and bad news about learning on the wards. The good news is that if you followed our study strategy for the preclinical years, you'll be on sound footing. During the clinical year you'll be focusing on diagnosis, management, and treatment, but all this rests on the foundation of medical knowledge that you've built. To maintain this, you just need to stay up to date with your reviews.

The bad news is that the clinical year imposes a different set of time constraints than the classroom experience you're used to. Instead of sitting at class or at home for dedicated study time, you'll have clinical responsibilities throughout the day. Your schedule will be outside your control with very little dedicated study time. The key, then, is to maximize your use of whatever free time you do have.

Therefore, in this section, our strategy will diverge somewhat from the preclinical years. The same psychological principles still apply, of course – you're still working with the same brain. But we have to adapt our strategy to the time constraints and the material you're learning.

> "The clinical year imposes a different set of time constraints than the classroom experience you're used to."

## How to learn

In the *Acquire* chapter in the *Learning Method*, we showed you how to learn in well-controlled environments dedicated to learning, where we have long, uninterrupted blocks of time and defined objectives. This worked fine for the preclinical year. But on the wards, a lot of your learning happens in unstructured experiences. These experiences include learning on the wards, learning from the encounters you have with patients, residents, and attendings. It also includes clinical simulations, conferences, seminars, and workshops.

We need to adapt and try to glean as much value as we can. The challenge here is capturing what we learn and getting it into our trusted learning system, Anki.

Although these experiences are diverse, the same principles of learning and memory apply, and so do the core tenets of our learning system. But the whole process is not going to be as neat as it is with dedicated study time. In any of these scenarios, the major challenges are to pay attention, have a framework to make sense of the incoming information, and capture the useful facts in a secure place for later review.

## Pay attention

Giving full attention to whatever is in front of us is a prerequisite for learning. This might seem obvious. But take a look around the next time you're on the wards or at a conference, and see how many people are dividing their attention between their iPhones, the people walking by, or even the fly in the room. In the modern world, we're surrounded by distractions that compete for our attention. And so we need to be mindful of our need to focus. If we want to learn, and we need to minimize distractions. It's OK to use your critical filter to decide what's worth attending to – not all conferences are high yield for your learning. But when you do actually want to learn something, you need to focus, and that needs to be a conscious effort.

Here are some tips for maintaining attention:

**Turn off your mobile device**. Unless you use it for capturing information, which we'll talk about below.

**Block specific distractions**. Our tools can be double-edged swords. Laptops and tablets are perfect examples. They're invaluable for taking notes during classes and conferences, but they are also a constant temptation to divert our attention. Often we could see most of our classmates (and ourselves!) checking out ESPN, Facebook or YouTube during a lecture. This is a scourge of modern life. To prevent this, consider installing a 'blocker' program, such as Self-Control for Mac that puts a temporary block on certain websites and your email.

**Commit to asking a question**. Nobody likes that guy who asks questions in order to show off. But committing yourself to ask at least one question forces you to focus on what is in front of you. If a question is genuine, it can be illuminating both to the asker and those around him or her. Don't overdo it, but if something is important to you, you'll likely truly want to ask the speaker or whoever to explain further.

# Have a framework in mind

Just as with any other learning we do, we need to make sense of it information in order to learn it. Having a framework is even more important in unstructured learning scenarios precisely because the information comes in a more haphazard, unvarnished form. When you read a textbook, all the information is presented in an intentional and coherent way. But if you're on the wards, or in a small group or with friends, there isn't much predetermined organization of ideas. Therefore, the onus is on *you*, the learner, to filter the incoming stream of information and impose an organizational framework that makes sense.

For example, on your internal medicine rotation, you and your team will undoubtedly discuss multiple disease entities whenever you run through a differential diagnosis. Information about any one disease will be scattered and piecemeal. But if you use the illness framework (see the Pathology chapter for details), you can thoughtfully organize this information into a coherent whole. Rather than become disoriented as differential diagnoses fly fast and furious, you'll understand the logic of "compare and contrast" that's driving the conversation.

# Noting and capturing

In our more controlled learning events, all the information we care about is on the page or on the screen. There is no risk of it getting away. But when we're learning "live," nuggets of information are fleeting, and we need to capture them for later processing.

The most straightforward way to capture ideas is by taking notes, either on paper or digitally. You can use anything from a notepad to a robust electronic note-taking program, such as Evernote. The important thing is to get stuff down on record, quickly and easily, so that you can defer processing until later.

Not every fact needs to be memorized, of course, so it's important to exercise good judgment. Here are some of the criteria we use to decide what goes into our notes:

**Record facts that you can't look up easily**. If a resident or attending is doing a "brain dump" on you that sounds a lot like a page from <u>Pocket Medicine</u>, you should be respectful and listen, but you don't need to scribble everything you hear. You know where you can find that information later. If, on the other hand, your attending explains her reasoning for choosing to order Test A over Test B, or why she chose to give ampicillin over amoxicillin, *that* you should take note of, since it's unique and you won't find that in a book so easily. In other words, pearls of clinical judgement or the 'art' of medicine are excellent fodder for notes.

**Record facts you want to look up later.** Often, someone mentions something that you don't know about, but you don't want to stop the flow of rounds to ask a question. Instead of interrupting the flow, make a note to look up the concept later on. Indeed, we keep a separate part of our note pads just for this kind of thing, with a little checkbox next to the concept, so that at the end of the day we can come back and resolve our curiosity on all these points.

**Record facts you want to get into Anki.** Although Anki has a mobile version on nearly every platform, we found that it's too cumbersome to create flashcards on the fly. Therefore, what we suggest is that you first make notes about factoids that you want to remember, and at a later time, convert them into Anki on your computer.

Finally, taking notes isn't just about capturing medical information. Often, we want to record our *reactions* to something we see or hear. That is a different kind of note, and sometimes, it can be the most important. Indeed, the majority of the notes that we took on the wards were ideas and reflections about the experience of being on the wards. The clinical setting is rich in possibilities for innovation, research, and improvement. Keep a notepad handy to scribble down how you feel after seeing a patient, or an idea for a new device or product that comes after a patient encounter. This is a form of learning too, and we recommend that you use some method to capture these kinds of thoughts. Many people find that having a Word or Evernote file for "future ideas" (for research projects, products, etc.) can be helpful for capturing those thoughts while dealing with the reality of having little time to actually act on them during clinical rotations.

# Get it into Anki

Not everything needs to be memorized. Some things are best left externalized on notes that you can access when needed. But when it comes to important facts that we *do* want to remember, we have Anki to rely on. In the same way that you use your highlights (if reading) or notes (if watching video) to make Anki cards, go through your notes regularly and make flashcards of the important factoids. Get it into the system sooner than later, preferably within 24-48 hours.

# What to learn

In your preclinical years, you've learned about the normal function of the body, and how pathological processes occur. You'll find that you often outshine even the residents in terms of your knowledge of mechanisms of drugs and the biochemical backgrounds on disease. But what the clinical years (and residency) teach, is how to translate that knowledge into diagnosis, management, and treatment of these diseases.

# The disease framework

Of the learning method, the most valuable element here will be the illness framework we used for pathology. When you see patients, on the wards or on exams, the main question you're usually asked is to determine which of several similar diseases the patient has, and how to treat it. Therefore, just as in your pathology course, the general focus of your studying should be in differentiating similar diseases, rather than diving directly into the minutiae of each disease. And the clinical years give you plenty of opportunity to practice that skill.

# Physical exam

The clinical year is also a time to hone your physical exam skills. You'll be seeing patients each day, and will have a multitude of opportunities to perform physical exams. Now is the time to build a strong physical exam toolkit you can use throughout your career. You can work your way through Bates' Guide to Physical Exam and History Taking as a guide to skills to build. Another great resource is JAMA's Rational Clinical Examination, which your school likely has an online subscription for. This resource highlights the evidence-based supports for each part of the clinical exam, so you can learn not only *what* to do but also *why* we do it. You'll also develop a deeper appreciation for what parts of the physical exam are truly important for honing in on diagnosis, and which are relatively lower yield.

# Learning for shelf exams

For better or worse, your grades on these clinical rotations are very important for residency applications. Most residency directors rank clinical grades as the number two (or sometimes even number one) consideration in choosing candidates. Schools vary greatly in how they determine your clinical grades, but the two largest components are your evaluations by the residents and attendings you're working with, and the shelf exam.

## Question-based studying

Because of the importance of your clinical grades, and therefore of the shelf exam, you may have to change our earlier focus on studying on boards and for life. For many of you looking to apply to competitive residencies, it is worth cramming a little to ensure you score well on board exams, rather than shoot purely for long-term retention.

To do that, you'll want to do practice questions. Questions are far more important for shelf exam preparation than studying from textbooks. To do well on shelf exams it's not enough to know the material; it's also necessary to know *how* the test makers tend to ask these questions. There tend to be key buzzwords and presentations that are predictably emphasized on exams, and it's as important to have a good feel for these as it is to know clinical facts and minutiae.

## Resources

Fortunately, there are a variety of resources that offer questions for your shelf review. The best one, in our experience, is the UWorld Q-bank for Step 2 CK. It has questions in each of the subjects that your rotations will cover, and offer good coverage of the major diseases and presentations in each.

Each rotation also has its own set of textbooks and question books from many different book series. Your school may have a program through the library allowing you to borrow books as necessary for each rotation. Unfortunately, while there are many series of review books to choose from, there is no clear winner. Each series has its strengths and weaknesses and even within the same series, quality varies widely by rotation. It's worth reaching out to upperclassmen, or even searching online forums, to see what previous students recommended for study resources. But again, the overall strategy is to use the textbooks to learn the content, but focus your energy primarily on doing questions to acquaint yourself with likely test practices.

# Anki

Anki remains a very powerful tool on the wards. During rotations, you do have a fair amount of downtime, but it comes at unpredictable intervals that may not allow you to sit down with a textbook to study. Anki's usefulness comes from its mobility, allowing you to get some productive studying done in these scattered bits of free time. Instead of spending that downtime bored and waiting around for something to happen, you can seize the opportunity to learn.

> "Anki's usefulness comes from its mobility, allowing you to get some productive studying done in these scattered bits of free time."

Despite its utility, we recommend that you use Anki mainly for *reviewing* material from the preclinical years, rather than maintaining all the knowledge that you're picking up on each clinical rotation. Rather than going through your clinical review books and putting all those facts into Anki, you'll have to use a light touch and only add the highest-yield facts that you've picked up.

Why is this? It's true that you could use Anki for retaining all the clinical knowledge you are acquiring on the wards. But recall that the major determinants of your grades on the wards are clinical evaluations from your residents and your attendings, along with your shelf exam score. Neither of these factors particularly benefit from using Anki for your clinical knowledge. In the limited time you have on rotations, creating a ton of new Anki cards is a luxury you can't afford. In fact, there's a danger that your evaluations may suffer if you're always glued to your iPhone. In an ideal world we could focus on long-term learning, but the reality is that we have to accommodate these constraints to protect our clinical grades.

As a result, we recommend that you use Anki mainly to review preclinical material, and only cautiously add important new material if time allows. This will allow you to consolidate your learning, make use of all the chunks of free time, while still making a good impression on the wards.

# Epilogue – The Future of Medicine

## Chapter 23: Becoming a 21st Century Doctor

# Chapter 23:
## Becoming A 21st Century Doctor

No matter what specialty you choose, you won't be practicing the kind of medicine that your professors in medical school are preparing you for. This shouldn't surprise you. After all, recognizably modern medicine is less than 100 years old. Penicillin was only discovered in 1928, and the vast majority of pharmaceuticals and treatments today were developed even more recently. Surgery goes back a little further, but it still likely did more harm than good until the mid-1800s, when hand-washing and other disinfection methods became common. Healers of some sort have a long history in every culture, and the skills of talking to patients and comforting them will never fall out of fashion. But the practice of modern medicine really has a very short history, and to be in medicine is to accept change as a way of life.

Medical schools, though, largely focus on producing students who will be able to function as good residents and doctors in today's world. That's important – we do have to be able to function as good residents. But it's not everything you'll need to learn to flourish in your career.

Determining what you *do* need to learn is a mild exercise in fortune-telling, which is definitely *not* an evidence-based endeavor. The best we can do is look at trends in medicine, and see what forward-looking practicing doctors are learning or wish they had learned. That said, here are some thoughts on the changes in medicine that are coming our way, and some of the skills it might take to become a 21st century doctor.

# The Business Landscape of Medicine Is Changing

One story that's always on the news is the political debate over whether the US should have a formally national healthcare system. This is an important question, and its results will shape the way we practice medicine. But it's only one of the many changes that the business of medicine is going to go through in our lifetimes. Payers – insurance and Medicare – are increasingly emphasizing metrics that are intended to track quality of care. Healthcare systems are consolidating as many private practices and independent hospitals are joining up with large hospital chains. At the same time, innovative practice models, from Accountable Care Organizations (ACOs) to cash-only practices are beginning to take off.

As a physician it's tempting to say that all this stuff is for businessmen, and that we should just worry about being clinicians. But changes in the business landscape affect the way we can practice medicine. Working for a consolidated hospital group involves different challenges than managing your own practice. Changes in what payers will pay for will influence what treatments you prescribe and how much time you can spend with each patient. Understanding the business of medicine will help you navigate the institutions you work in to deliver best care to your patients. And for the entrepreneurially minded, it's vital to understand how medical practices work in order to strike out and practice medicine the way you want.

There are two major ways to go about a career in medicine: you can be the employee of a hospital or other large healthcare system, or you may join a private practice. A 2012 Accenture report showed that 39% of doctors operated in private practices, compared to 61% who are employed by other organizations. How you choose to practice will influence just how much business knowledge you need to have.

At the minimum, if you know for sure that you want to work for a hospital, it's important to understand the economics of medicine. If you understand how healthcare payment works, how hospitals get paid by Medicare, Medicaid, and private insurance, you can better understand why hospitals work the way they do, and why they try to influence physicians to practice medicine in certain ways that are best for the organization's bottom line. You can also better understand your patients' behavior – why they may or may not be willing to take medications as prescribed, and whether clinic visits and paying for drugs poses a financial strain that makes it hard for them to do what's medically best for them. And given the controversy over the cost of healthcare, it's worth familiarizing yourself with how much various tests and procedures cost. These are not things that medical schools cover in much depth. According to a 2011 paper, less than a quarter of internal medicine residents and attendings were able to even vaguely estimate charges for diagnostic tests at their hospital. But they did say that they were eager to learn more, and being in medical school, you're in a great position to get that information earlier.

If you are interested in potentially doing private practice, the bar becomes higher. Most residencies don't give in-depth training on the business aspects of running a practice, so you'll have to learn the fundamentals on your own. Worthwhile topics include basic accounting for small businesses, the major legal matters in setting up medical practice, and the basics of marketing. Even if you're not sure that you're going into private practice, a little understanding of these topics can be helpful, if only to demystify the process. Many doctors consider doing private practice, whether to try out a new practice model or to move to a rural area and help the underserved, but are intimidated by all the required knowledge that they didn't get a chance to learn in medical school and residency. By forearming yourself with that knowledge now, you give yourself a chance to make that decision freely and be able to choose how practice medicine in a way you find rewarding.

# Technology Is Changing the Role of the Physician

Doctors used to diagnose and treat patients with no more reference material than an old textbook and some back issues of medical journals sitting in a file cabinet. That has clearly changed. Now that we have computers and smartphones that can bring the latest information on diagnosis and treatment to our fingertips. At the same time, computers, such as IBM's Watson, have made impressive strides towards being able to diagnose illnesses as well as humans, given a set of symptoms.

What does this all mean for us? Most prosaically, it means that we don't need to just be memorizing machines. A lot of medical school emphasizes the amount of information we have in our heads. But in practice, any time we need to look something up, we'll have the tools at hand to look up the latest clinical guidelines. This doesn't mean that medical school is worthless. On the contrary, having this volume of information at hand only makes it more important to have a basic map of knowledge in our heads, so we can make sense of it. But it means that instead of trying to memorize everything, we should be generating frameworks for thinking about the topics we're learning, in the knowledge that we can look up more detail if necessary. For example, it may not be necessary to memorize all the side effects of ACE inhibitors, but what's important is that we know that they can cause angioedema and cough, and where to look up the rest of the rarer side effects on Epocrates.

But also, as computers perform some of the specialized knowledge functions of MDs, our role is increasingly to synthesize information and lead healthcare teams. The increasing role of mid-level providers such as physician's assistants and nurse practitioners will only reinforce this trend. We won't just be data banks making mundane treatment decisions. Rather, we'll delegate some tasks to other healthcare workers, assimilate the information they've gathered, and lead the team in executing a plan. In this environment, "soft skills" – leadership, communication, and public speaking, will be needed for us to perform this role well.

At the same time, while computers may eventually be able to perform diagnosis *given the patient's symptoms*, it still falls on the physician to be an expert gatherer of clinical information. Interviewing skills – the ability to develop rapport with a patient and elicit their symptoms and all their other relevant information, will be at a premium. Physical exam skills will remain important as well.

Finally, medical research, whether in basic-science advances such as medical imaging and genomics or the high-stakes world of clinical trials, is becoming increasingly quantitative. So basic statistical literacy will be a must for us to keep abreast of, and critically evaluate, the new research that will change our practice during our careers. For those of us interested in performing research, an in-depth grounding in statistics and data analysis will be important.

# New Opportunities to Advance the Role of Technology

These changes in medical practice will be scary. Some skills – notably the pure memorization aspect of medicine – will become less valuable. And there's a temptation to fight against these changes as dangerous to doctors' professional status and standard of living.

But this is not quite the lesson of history. You may have heard the term "Luddite" used to describe late adopters of technology. The term comes from the original Luddites – English textile workers who smashed looms, fearful of the risk that mechanical looms posed to their jobs. But in fact the Industrial Revolution that the looms presaged ultimately raised living standards for workers of all skill levels. Similarly, the assembly line, which seemed to threaten the livelihood of factory workers, ultimately led to the higher wages that skilled mechanical workers enjoyed by the mid-20th century.

In each case the logic was this: technological change hurt those who competed directly with machines, but massively helped workers who could work *with* the machines. If you could maintain a loom or maintain a welding machine, mechanization would work for you, not against you. The same is likely to happen in medicine.

So what does working *with* emerging medical technology look like? Specializing in roles that computers cannot fill – like leadership, communication, and knowledge organization – is one way. Another is to have the skills to be at the forefront of changing technology. Instead of adapting to technology, you can help drive its evolution.

It's true that a lot of the people working with technology have heavily specialized skillsets – whether in programming, engineering, or entrepreneurship. We're doctors first and foremost, and we're not trying to become hackers. But often, what these technologists need is our experience in all things medical. They don't have in-depth knowledge of how doctors' workflows work, or how patients tend to make healthcare decisions – exactly the skills that we've spent years developing. And they need this knowledge to figure out what problems are out there to be solved, and how to target their products to doctors and patients. So one way doctors can help pioneer new technology is being the "medical expert" who can communicate with the technologists and help make decisions about what problems in medicine are worth attacking.

For that, you don't need to be an expert in technology, but you have to be able to speak the language. You have to know what computers can and cannot do. You have to know what engineering challenges are hard, and which are easy. And you should have some sense of what technological approaches to medicine have been tried in the past, and which succeeded and which failed.

There's a few approaches to cultivating this knowledge. One is simply to talk to your computer science and engineering friends from college or elsewhere, sharing the problems that you and they are working on. In this way you may both get a sense of what the major challenges are in each other's fields. A more proactive approach might be to learn a little bit about coding on your own. This could be very simple and doesn't necessarily need a huge time commitment. The goal is to get an idea of how programmers see the world, and what computers are good at doing as well as what they find challenging. Finally, you can follow the news around health technologies. A few years of tracking what the hot fields are, and seeing the rise and fall of different technologies, could give you both a working familiarity with major trends in health technology as well as a deeper sense of what people are working on and what it takes to succeed in health technology.

# Create Your Own Future

In this book we've taught you how to study more effectively, to do more long-term learning in less time. Certainly, it's valuable to learn more and be more knowledgeable in our clinical practice. But the other benefit of learning *efficiently* is that it lets us take some time *away* from learning, towards developing other complementary skills. The world needs knowledgeable doctors, but even more than that, it needs doctors who practice medicine humanistically, and doctors who think carefully about how the future is evolving and work hard to create the future of medicine that they want to see.

We hope that with these tools in hand, you exceed all your academic expectations for medical school and residency. Equally, we hope that you take this opportunity to become well-rounded as a physician. But most of all, we hope you take this spirit of experimentation – of deciding what you want to accomplish, then *doing* it, no matter what the conventional wisdom is – into the rest of your careers. The future of medicine is not set in stone, it's something we decide with the choices we make in our careers. Let's make it a good one.

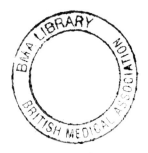

Made in the USA
Charleston, SC
10 January 2016